DATE DUE			
Apr 5 '76			
May 16 '77 E			
Nov 23 '77			
Feb 16 79			
Apr 25 '80			
Nov 8 '80			
Feb 10 '81			

Books by Dewey Schurman

ATHLETIC FITNESS   1975

VOLLEYBALL   1974

ATHLETIC FITNESS

ATHLETIC

ATHENEUM   1975   NEW YORK

Dewey Schurman

FITNESS

The Athlete's Guide to Training and Conditioning

Acknowledgments

THIS BOOK would not have been possible without the help of some very busy people who found the time to discuss the various aspects of athletic training. I would particularly like to thank Jim Bush of UCLA, Chuck Krpata and Frank Egenhoff of the San Francisco 49ers, Gary Tuthill of the Los Angeles Rams, and Dr. John H. K. Vogel of the Santa Barbara Heart & Lung Institute.

A special thanks is due to photographers Bob Ponce and Rafael Maldonado, and to Gus Mee, member of the U.S. volleyball team for the 1973 World Games in Moscow and coach of the nationally ranked volleyball team of the University of California at Santa Barbara, who served as the model for most of the exercises illustrated in this book.

The cover photograph of the Rams stretching during a pregame warm-up is by Bob Ponce; the photograph of top California distance runner Eric Hulst was taken by Burt Davis, Jr.

Contents

vii

ATHLETIC FITNESS

Introduction

THIS BOOK was written for athletes, and the more important sports and athletic activities are in your life, the more valuable it can be for you.

The training and conditioning methods outlined in this book are those practiced by today's top professional and amateur athletes, and for the serious athlete these techniques not only should help improve athletic performance, but can even make the difference between a successful career in sports and a career cut short by injury.

But you do not have to be a fulltime or career athlete to benefit from the conditioning programs presented in the following pages. Even the weekend athlete will find advice for making limited exer-

3

cise time more worthwhile, as well as common sense guidance for weight control, for easing post-weekend aches and pains, and for reducing risk of injury in athletic activities.

In short, no matter what your sport, level of competition, or athletic ambitions, if you are willing to find the time and make the effort, these programs can help you get in shape—and stay in shape.

BEFORE YOU START

Physical fitness does not come overnight.

Common sense should tell you that you should not begin a strenuous exercise or conditioning program (or athletic activity) without first gradually building up to the level of effort involved.

Before starting any physical fitness program, you should see your doctor and have a physical examination.

However, an ordinary physical examination may not be enough.

A test administered to most professional athletes is the exercising electrocardiogram or "stress EKG."

The normal electrocardiogram is the standard

test for any possible heart irregularities. However, the heart undergoes much more stress during physical exercise, and a stress EKG, taken during exercise, is much more likely to pick up any warning signal than the normal EKG, given while the subject is resting.

A stress EKG (usually conducted while the subject is pedaling a stationary bicycle or walking-running on a treadmill) under the supervision of a physician is recommended for any fulltime athlete or anyone in any of the following categories:

1. Over thirty years old
2. More than 15 pounds overweight
3. History of heart trouble in the immediate family (parents, brother or sister)
4. Beginning an exercise program and not already physically active, or stepping up to a more intense level of training or competition
5. Heavy smoker, high blood pressure, or personal history of serious or chronic illness.

1. The Basics

✦ He never could accept anything less than a maximum effort—and that included practices too. He would say, "If you can't take my pressure then for sure you can't take it in a game." He could rip you in those practices. I know there were many times when I was just as nervous—more sometimes—going to practice as playing in a game. And it worked. On third-and-ten in a close game, in a championship game, you really believed you could do it.

BOYD DOWLER, *Green Bay Packers*

✦ He pushed you to the end of your endurance and then beyond it. And if there was a reserve there, well, he found that, too.

HENRY JORDAN, *Green Bay Packers*

W H A T   I S   "getting in shape"?

In football a few years back, when Vince Lombardi was coaching the Packers, it meant wind sprints across the field, calisthenics and playing into shape during training camp and practices.

Times change.

Jim Bush, who has coached world record runners in track at UCLA and has helped top professional athletes in football, basketball, hockey, and tennis with their conditioning programs, calls wind sprints "dangerous" and says they are about the worst training method a team can use.

Calisthenics, the "jumping jacks" and "herky-jerky toe touchers" that are still a key feature of many exercise programs, have been dropped entirely by several professional teams, including the Los Angeles Rams and San Francisco 49ers, and replaced instead by slow "stretching" exercises.

Playing into shape? In professional sports today, where most careers last only a couple of years, the athlete who is not in shape at the beginning of the season may find out the hard way that there is always someone waiting to take his place if he slows down, is injured, or cannot keep going at full strength for an entire game or season.

Year-round training has long been an accepted fact of life in such sports as track and swimming, where endurance and conditioning are often more important than natural talent or ability. But the notion has spread to other sports in recent years, with more and more athletes, coaches, and trainers realizing that a balanced, year-round conditioning program improves performance and reduces injuries.

In competitive athletics, where players and coaches are always looking for that "winning edge," physical conditioning may mean the difference between winning a game and losing it, or between a great season and a disastrous one.

Dodger great Maury Wills once recognized that there are baseball players who make it to the major leagues on sheer natural ability and others who may lack some of the physical gifts such as size (like Wills) or speed but make it anyway through determination and hard work. But, as Wills noted, it is only those few players who combine natural skills with hard work who earn the label "superstar."

Some naturally gifted athletes get by on talent alone for most of their careers—through high school, where they were the best players on the team, and maybe even in college. But sooner or later, nearly every athlete finds a level of competition to meet his skills.

Jim Bush has told football players who have come to him after being drafted by a professional team that having been the best athlete on their college football teams won't help when they start playing against other football greats in the pro ranks.

"I tell them," he says, "when you go into training camp, you will have to be in the greatest shape of your life, and that's not something you can do in just a few weeks."

There is a world of difference between basic physical fitness necessary for good health (which, studies indicate, many Americans fail even to approach) and the level of physical fitness required for top-class athletic competition.

But the elements of fitness are the same for both levels.

Athletic ability includes several factors (among them, agility, balance, coordination, quickness, speed, and timing), but the three elements that are essential to fitness, and the three that can be developed and improved most through training and conditioning are *endurance, flexibility,* and *strength.*

These three elements are fundamental to athletic fitness. Conditioning in these areas will also lead to improvements in other areas, such as quickness and speed, and the athlete who ignores or neglects any one of the three is likely to pay for it either in performance or with an injury.

The conditioning programs described in this book center on endurance, flexibility, and strength, and can be adapted to virtually any level of athletic fitness, including that required in such sports as professional football, basketball, and tennis.

But as Los Angeles Ram trainer Gary Tuthill

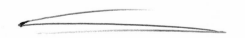

points out, "You can have the greatest conditioning program in the world, but if the individual athlete doesn't work at it, it's worthless."

With that in mind, let's take a look at what it takes to get in shape.

2. Endurance

Fatigue makes cowards of us all.
VINCE LOMBARDI

The professional coach is an expert in his field. Nobody knows his sport, whether it is football, basketball, or whatever, better than he does. But not many pro coaches know how to get an athlete physically ready to play. . . . And not many athletes know either.
JIM BUSH, *UCLA track coach*

E N D U R A N C E or stamina is the ability of the body to keep going, to withstand fatigue and continue its exertion or activity.

It is the area of physical fitness that coaches usually concentrate on when players arrive in training camp, and it is the area that they continue to stress in practices throughout the season.

Endurance is the obvious factor in the performance of the marathon runner or the long distance swimmer but, although less apparent, it is a key in-

11

gredient in virtually every sport.

In football and basketball, the team that comes from behind to win in the last quarter is usually the team in the best condition—that is, the team with the most endurance. That was the lesson Lombardi preached over and over again to his players during practice.

UCLA's John Wooden always expected his basketball players to be in better shape than any team they faced, saying that with two closely matched teams the game is usually decided in the last minutes, when conditioning is the big factor. Time-outs, he said, are usually determined by a team's physical condition. He always wanted his team to benefit from the time-outs called by the other team when it was tired, saving the UCLA time-outs for strategic purposes.

Even less physically demanding sports such as baseball and golf have elements of endurance. The pitcher who begins to lose his stuff and tire in the late innings and the golfer who plays well on the front nine but watches his score soar on the back nine are both often suffering from a lack of endurance.

And even many injuries can be traced to poor endurance conditioning. If an athlete tires, he must strain to keep going, and it is when an athlete is straining that he is most likely to pull a muscle. As fatigue increases, so do injuries. Football injuries, for example, occur most often late in a game or near the end of a practice.

When you are tired, you also are not as sharp physically or mentally as when you are fresh; and that may mean not being able to get out of the way of a runner trying to break up a double play if you are a shortstop, or not even seeing a crackback block coming if you are a linebacker.

The problem with trying to "play into shape" is that most sports (including baseball, basketball, football, tennis, and volleyball) are stop-and-start activities that do not provide the sustained, non-stop exercise that builds endurance.

To build endurance, you must exercise hard enough and long enough to force your body's respiratory (breathing) and cardiovascular (heart and blood vessel) systems to deliver greater amounts of oxygen-carrying blood to your muscles and tissues—and keep delivering it for some time.

Muscular fatigue is basically the result of an inadequate supply of oxygen. As endurance increases, the circulatory system becomes more efficient in its delivery of oxygen (in the blood) throughout the body, allowing muscles to retain

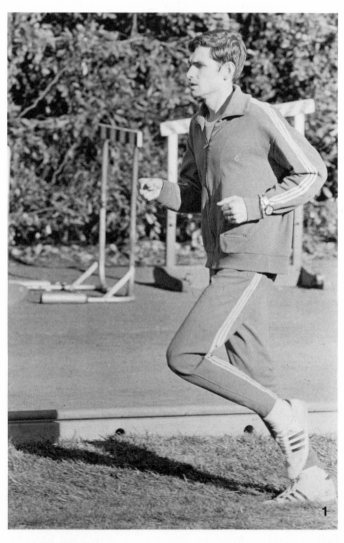

Jim Ryun, world-record holder in the mile, demonstrates his relaxed running style during a training workout. (PHOTO: BOB PONCE)

maximum strength longer, to forestall fatigue, and even to inhibit stress and illness.

It stands to reason that you cannot develop your endurance reserves if you do not push your body past those early feelings of tiredness and fatigue.

One measure of circulatory efficiency is the maximum amount of oxygen the body can take in and use, known as *maximal oxygen uptake*. The test for this, usually given on a treadmill, measures the amount of oxygen consumed by the body in milliliters of oxygen per kilogram of body weight per minute.

While the healthy average person may have a score in the low 40s, the scores among well-conditioned athletes may range from the mid 50s to the high 70s. However, former mile record holder Jim Ryun has been measured at between 83 and 85!

Running has long been recognized as the best endurance builder for athletes (except for swimmers, who naturally rely on swimming); for most serious athletes, "getting in shape" means running.

Four years ago, Los Angeles Laker guard Gail Goodrich went to Jim Bush and told the UCLA track coach that he wanted to be able to start the approaching NBA season as fast as he usually ended it (after playing himself into shape) and not slow down at all during the season.

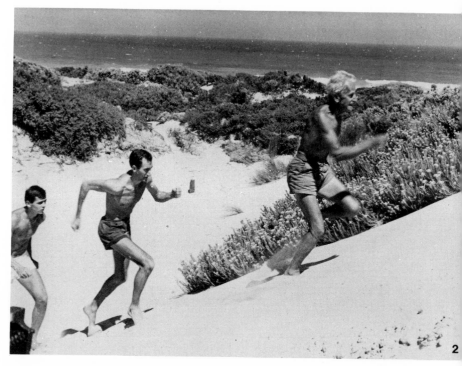

2

Percy Cerutty, shown leading former world-record miler Herb Elliott up a sand hill during a training session in Australia, revolutionized modern conditioning techniques by having his athletes, including Elliott and John Landy, train with weights and do much of their running up hills.

Bush devised a running program that Goodrich has continued ever since, crediting it to a large degree for his increased quickness and endurance and his emergence as one of the league's top scorers.

Kathy May, a young tennis professional, found running not only increased her endurance but made her quicker. After months on the Bush-designed running program, which included running up hills near UCLA, she found she was getting to balls she had been unable to reach with her racquet before. (Arthur Ashe and Roscoe Tanner are two other top tennis pros who turned to a running coach to increase their quickness on the courts.)

The key to the Bush program is learning how to run relaxed at a fast pace.

Relaxed running does not mean jogging.

Too many people, Bush says, go out and "jog" a mile or two and end up hurting their knees and joints from the continual pounding. A fast but relaxed one-mile run is far better for your body than a slow but hard-pounding jog of two or three miles.

"The athletes who are willing to work hard to learn how to relax at a fast tempo will be the best athletes," Bush says.

Such training does not happen overnight.

It takes a minimum of six to eight weeks to build what Bush calls the "base" or foundation for conditioning. But the athlete who can learn to discipline himself and train for that length of time will be able to take any drill a coach can throw at him in practice—and with less chance of injury, according to Bush.

Relaxed running begins in the face.

"If your jaw is clenched, you can't be relaxed," Bush says. So over and over again he tells his runners to let their jaws "flop" or "bounce."

Another sign of tightness is hunched shoulders. Let them drop while you run, he advises.

Instead of clenching your fists while you run, put your thumb on your forefinger; it will help you keep your hands, arms, and shoulders relaxed.

As you run, try to find a pace that feels *relaxing* to you: If it seems too slow, speed up slightly; if it feels too fast, slow down a bit. Then, each day try to run either a little faster or a little farther.

Bush, who usually advises his nontrack athletes to start out running five days a week around a large playing field near the UCLA track (about a 1,000-yard run), says that running a greater distance each time may do a little more for the respiratory system but, depending on the athlete, "you will probably get about the same results both ways."

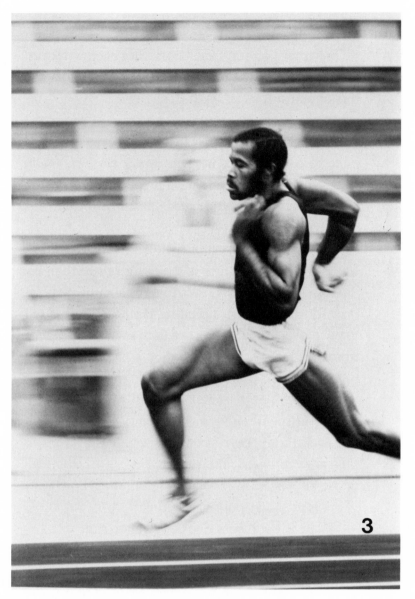

3

A world-class runner, Lee Evans, shows the combination of strength and relaxation necessary for top running performance.

Whether you run faster or farther each workout, each week you'll find that you will be able to run faster and still be relaxed, Bush says.

Even an O. J. Simpson doesn't run at top speed all the time, Bush notes. If he did, he wouldn't be able to cut. Instead, he *runs under control,* ready to stop or cut. It's only when he breaks into the clear that he "turns the speed valve open" and runs at full speed.

The danger with wind sprints in practice, Bush says, is that the runner is straining rather than relaxing. And straining leads to muscle pulls. Several pro football teams, including the Rams, now tell their players to *stride* rather than sprint in practice for that reason.

"Train, but don't strain" is the most important phrase in athletics, according to Bush.

If you spend enough time running, you will almost certainly have occasions when you seem to find a *rhythm* in your running, when it seems almost effortless, or as if you're running downhill: That is relaxed running.

There is not just one correct way to run.

"John Smith [world record holder for the 440] had the most beautiful form of any athlete I've ever seen, but if a runner tried to copy that form, he would probably tie up," Bush said. Wayne Collett (silver medalist at the 1972 Olympics), he added, was not a classic or "picture" runner, "but he ran what was relaxed to him."

Another advocate of relaxed running is Bud Winter, former San Jose State track coach whose sprinters dominated world track records in the 1960s. He says that a runner runs fastest at four-fifths effort.

Just as the baseball player concentrating on a nice, easy swing sometimes hits the ball hard, but pops it up or misses it entirely when he swings for the fence, the athlete who can learn to increase his effort *while remaining relaxed* is bound to improve his skills—whether those skills are hitting a baseball or golfball, high-jumping or running.

Still, without endurance, even improved skills are incomplete.

Bush points out that it is not always the fastest runner who wins the race. The fastest sprinter may pull up halfway down the track with a pulled hamstring muscle.

Even a 100-yard dash requires endurance. If two runners have the same speed, the one who maintains his best form from start to finish will win. If one is slightly faster but is out of shape, his muscles will start to fatigue earlier; and if he loses his form in the last few yards of the race, the other runner may just beat him to the tape.

The basic Bush running program consists of starting with a fast-but-relaxed run of from one-half mile to 1,000 yards, trying to run slightly faster or slightly farther each workout, five days a week for a minimum of six to eight weeks.

A minimum program for staying in shape year round, according to Bush, is a one-mile run at a striding (about three-fourth speed) pace, three times a week. If you are running a mile in about eight minutes, try to cut that time down to seven, six, or even five minutes, Bush says.

If you are training for a sport that involves running *speed* (baseball, basketball, football, soccer), allow for at least eight weeks of running before the start of practices. Then, in the last four weeks before practices, start working on your speed by running up hills and doing shorter (40 to 50 yard) "striding" runs.

At UCLA, members of the track team tackle the Hill—a 508-yard, strength-sapping course that gradually steepens to about a 30-degree slope. It is a torturous climb that has caused more than one member of the track team to lose his lunch, but Bruin runners including Smith and Collett credit the Hill with building the strength and endurance that helped them become world-class quarter-milers.

Bush advises his runners to try the Hill at half or three-quarter speed, and to stop whenever their legs *start* to tighten up—even if they are only half-way up the Hill.

Many runners fail to make it to the top of the Hill, even after several tries. But for his track squad, which starts training in September, Bush sets a goal of five runs to the top a day, three days a week, by Christmas.

Although the Hill at UCLA has become relatively famous in the last year (so much so that the grassy path has been worn completely down to dirt and Bush prefers not to disclose its location to joggers), the Bruin coach says that any hill will do the job. He himself picked up the idea while in New Zealand several years ago, where local runners trained on a half-mile hill run.

If hills are not available, it is usually possible to find a nearby football stadium where you can run up the stadium steps.

But whether you run hills or stadium steps, Bush advises against running or even jogging back down, and recommends instead simply walking back down.

A basic benefit of a running program is increased *quickness*—that ability to move quickly forward, backwards and laterally. Pro football teams don't worry too much about the speed of an interior lineman (guard, tackle, center), but professional coaches do look for quickness in all their prospects. It is a characteristic the Rams call "happy feet."

"Speed is either there or not there," Bush says, "but quickness can be increased by developing leg strength—and that means running."

TRAINING NOTES

1. Warming up is a prerequisite for any exercise, including running. Before running, do some leg- and back-stretching exercises, and then do a slow jog for a minute or two before actually starting to run.

2. When possible, do your running on grass. Running on a hard surface such as cement or asphalt is much harder on your legs and joints. On the coasts, some runners like to exercise on the beach. However, it is important to run on relatively flat sand, because running on a sloping beach can cause hip strain. If, like world-class sprinter Steve Williams, you also run in soft beach sand as a con-

ditioner, get used to it gradually or your calf muscles will probably tie up or cramp.

3. Money spent on a good running shoe is one of the best investments a serious athlete can make. A cheap or bad-fitting pair of shoes not only makes running uncomfortable but can lead to a wide range of serious leg, foot, and hip injuries. A good training shoe has a much heavier sole than a sole used in competition. A good example is the SL-72 by Adidas, according to Bush.

4. One of the best substitutes for running is rope skipping. Timewise, it is at least the equal of running as an endurance conditioner. Vince Lombardi used to recommend it to his football players for developing better footwork and agility, while boxers have relied on it for years for the same reasons. Golfer Gary Player and tennis star Stan Smith also skip rope to stay in shape.

5. Many professional coaches encourage their players to find some sport they like (tennis, basketball, handball) to help stay in shape during the off season. There can be other benefits in such activity. Johnny Robinson, Kansas City Chief safety, credits tennis with helping him learn to back pedal and move laterally—movements critical to success in his football position on defense.

6. Europeans first developed two endurance

training methods now widely used in the United States—interval training and circuit training.

In *interval training,* an athlete will run a series of fast runs of 50 to 440 yards or more, interrupted only by brief, walk-jog, "rest periods." The idea is to develop the ability of the body's respiratory and cardiovascular systems to recover quickly from fatigue and to increase the body's ability to cope with the muscular fatigue that comes with "oxygen debt"—the system's inability to supply oxygen rapidly to all parts of the body during extended exercise.

The Rams use a typical interval program in their workouts once a week: Each receiver and defensive back runs *at a striding pace* 440 yards once, 330 yards twice, 220 yards three times, and 110 yards four times, with a two-minute rest between runs and a very slow 880-yard "cool down" at the end.

Sherman Chavoor, who helped coach Mark Spitz, Debbie Meyer, and Mike Burton to world swimming records, developed an intensive interval program in which he cut resting periods between full-speed swims from several minutes down to one minute, to 30 seconds, and finally down to just 10 seconds between swims. During the training, Chavoor said, swimmers not only increased their bodys' ability to make the best use of its oxygen, but actually began building up and storing certain enzymes in the muscles that would allow them to continue to work without oxygen.

In *circuit* training, the athlete completes a series of exercises (push-ups, sit-ups, chin-ups, rope skipping, parallel bar dips) as a "circuit," with no rest between exercises, and then repeats the circuit once or twice more, each time doing the maximum number of each exercise that he can do in one minute.

7. How much is *too much* exercise? If fatigue lasts more than two hours after the exercise, the workout is generally considered to have been too vigorous. Another check is your pulse rate. If after 10 minutes following the end of your workout your pulse rate is still over 100, it was probably too strenuous.

Overtraining is a case of too much exercise over a period of time. It is necessary for any athlete to build up gradually to strenuous exercise workouts, and even world-class athletes sometimes fall victim to too much training. A few common signs of overtraining are: inability to stay asleep, increased clumsiness or poor coordination, poor appetite, and fatigue occurring earlier in workouts.

Overtraining most often occurs in athletes training for endurance events such as distance running, but it can happen to anyone who pushes his body far beyond the limits to which it has become accustomed. The cure is relatively simple: rest, and cut back on workouts until symptoms are gone.

8. Just as it is necessary to warm up before any exercise, it is also important to have a "cooling down" period. After any run, you should walk-jog at a very slow pace for at least five minutes to allow the blood (that has been delivered to your arms and legs to meet the overload demands of exercise) to return to your heart and brain. If you don't cool down after strenuous exercise, you are risking the chance of a dizzy spell or fainting.

That is one reason why, at any track meet, a runner who finishes a race will walk around (even if he has to lean on someone to do it).

Another reason is to ease aches and pains the following day. An accumulation of lactic acid in the muscles, due to a lack of oxygen being supplied to the muscle, contributes to muscular fatigue. A cooling down period allows that lactic acid buildup to partly dissipate. If the lactic acid buildup is not allowed to break down, muscles will be sorer and stiffer the next day. For that reason, the Los Angeles Rams players sometimes jump in a swimming pool for a few minutes after practice.

9. Although a minimum of six to eight weeks is required for an athlete to get in shape running, it takes only about three weeks for an athlete to lose that conditioning, according to Bush. This is one reason why a short vacation from training, or even a minor injury, can set an athlete's training schedule off by several weeks—yet another argument for staying in shape year round.

10. Even golfers, who probably take more long walks than any other athletes, worry about their endurance. Johnny Miller takes long hunting hikes through swampy lands near home to keep his legs in shape, while Hubert Green, another top money winner on the pro tour, jogs about a mile a day when he is not playing. Green, who says that strong legs are the most important thing physically in golf, adds that while most pro golfers don't talk too much about it, most jog to keep in shape.

11. Probably the most convenient test yet devised to gauge your endurance is the Air Force conditioning test developed by Dr. Kenneth Cooper.* The Los Angeles Rams are just one of several professional teams that advise their players to use the test to determine their endurance. The test itself simply involves running, jogging, and, if necessary, walking, for as far as possible in 12 minutes

* *The New Aerobics,* M. Evans & Co., New York, 1970.

around a quarter-mile track or some other pre-measured route. Your endurance is determined by the distance covered during the 12 minutes, as follows:

	RATING	DISTANCE COVERED
1.	Very poor	Less than 1.0 mile
2.	Poor	1.0 to 1.24 miles
3.	Fair	1.25 to 1.49 miles
4.	Good	1.50 to 1.74 miles
5.	Excellent	1.75 miles or more

3. Strength

If your muscles are strong, they will react quicker and won't fatigue as fast.

JIM BUSH

WEIGHT LIFTING was once considered harmful to athletes and left strictly to body builders. Now training with weights is accepted as a standard part of conditioning in almost every sport, from football to track and swimming.

Weight training, along with advances in coaching techniques, is one major reason why athletes are getting bigger, stronger, and faster each year, and why records are being broken at an ever faster clip.

Of course, weight training isn't necessary for every athlete. The strictly recreational, weekend athlete definitely needs both endurance and flexibility conditioning for his general health, but sel-

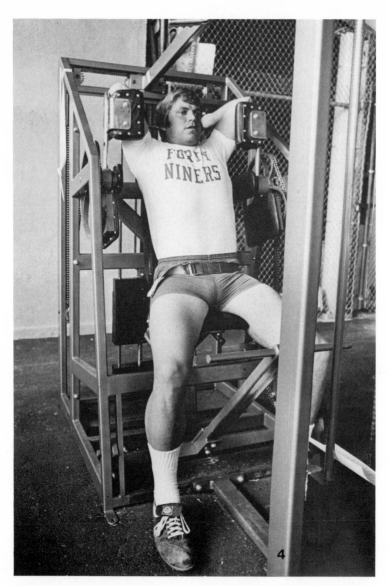

4

The key to success in any weight-training program is effort of the kind Jim Schnietz demonstrates while working out on a Nautilus weight machine during training camp with the San Francisco 49ers. (PHOTOS: RAFAEL MALDONADO)

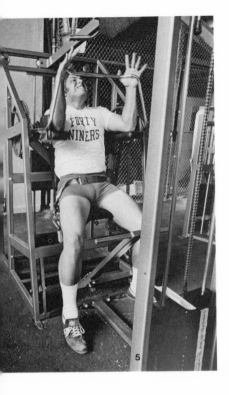

5

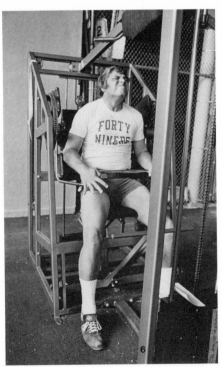

6

dom needs the strength gains that training with weights will produce.

On the other hand, if the weekend tennis player suffers from tennis elbow or a sore shoulder, weight training may be exactly what he needs to ease the ailment and make his sport more enjoyable (see Chapter 6).

It is generally not a good idea to begin training with weights at too early an age. Dr. Robert Kerlan, who acts as a consultant to many professional teams, including the Rams, Lakers, Kings, and Angels, recommends that any weight training begun while a youngster is still growing should be done only with very light weights to avoid putting excessive stress on the still-developing skeletal frame. The growth centers near the end of the bones, called epiphysis, can be seriously damaged by compression from lifting heavy weights during the growth years, Kerlan says.

But for the serious or fulltime athlete, the time and effort spent in weight training is well worthwhile, because in nearly every sport it is the strongest, most powerful athletes who are the most successful, just as in baseball it is the homerun hitter, not the singles hitter, who draws the biggest salary.

In some sports, such as football, weight training has become almost mandatory. Vince Lombardi once said, "Football is not a *contact* sport; dancing is a contact sport. Football is a hitting sport." In a game of collisions, weight training is one way a player can gain the size and strength he needs to keep from being overmatched physically, and as added protection against injury.

Another sport that has recently begun to place a strong emphasis on weight training is volleyball, which has become the latest entry in the professional sports world.

Volleyball is primarily a game of hitting and blocking at an eight-foot-high net. The taller player naturally has an advantage, but with weight training the smaller athlete can sometimes outjump a taller opponent. Gus Mee, who played on the U.S. volleyball team in the 1973 World Games in Moscow, stands 6–1. With weight training, he was able to increase his jump about 8 inches, so that he could touch a mark 11 feet high.

An extensive weight program was also credited as a major factor in the development of the Cuban national volleyball team, which, under Russian coaching, was transformed in just a few years from a rather ordinary team to a powerhouse that eliminated the U.S. national team during the 1972 Olympic qualifying rounds.

The Russians have long considered weight training as a key part of their training program for athletes in nearly every sport.

In this country, weight training has also been taken up by most track and field athletes, baseball players (including Reggie Jackson, Carl Yastrzemski, and 1974 Cy Young winner Mike Marshall), golfers (following the lead of South Africa's Gary Player), and swimmers. (Dr. James Counsilman, Indiana University and U.S. Olympic coach, recommends weight exercises to improve a swimmer's muscular endurance and speed.)

Basketball, which like volleyball requires strong jumping ability, is another sport in which athletes have turned to weight training as part of their conditioning.

Some basketball coaches, including John Wooden and the Lakers' Bill Sharman, have discouraged weight training for their players out of a concern it might affect their shooting touch. Other basketball coaches, however, advise their athletes to work on leg exercises that will help their jump, while recommending that they avoid arm and upper body exercises.

Gary Tuthill says he would encourage weight training for all sports. And Tuthill has worked with other athletes as well as football players; before he was a trainer with the Detroit Lions and the Rams, he was head trainer for all sports at USC for 11 years.

Weight training is neither weight lifting nor body building.

Weight lifting is a sport itself, in which the athlete's performance is judged by the amount of weight he can lift in a series of events. The actual lifting events vary in the two types of weight lifting competition, Olympic lifting and power lifting.

Still, it is the heavyweight- and superheavyweight-class lifters, some of them roly-poly behemoths weighing over 300 pounds, who are responsible for the common notion that weight lifting always adds unwanted bulk along with strength.

That's just not the case. To a degree, strength is determined by muscle size, but it isn't necessary for a player to gain weight and muscle bulk for a weight training program to be effective. And body builders, many of whom are not particularly strong for their size, have shown that increasing muscle size to maximum dimensions does not always produce the greatest strength.

In *body building,* weight training techniques are used as a means of increasing muscle size and definition as much as possible.

Of course, not everyone wants to look like a Mr.

Universe. But weight training won't produce a Mr. Universe body unless that is the specific goal of the individual. Most of the top body builders, such as Arnold Schwarzenegger (who at twenty-eight is generally recognized as the leading body builder in the world), work out several hours a day, six days a week, using training techniques quite different from those used in athletic weight training.

For example, when a body builder is working to maximize his muscular definition—the sharply individualized muscles that are a primary consideration in judging body building contests—he increases both the speed of his workout exercises and the number of times he does each exercise. In athletic weight training, the technique is often just the opposite—work slowly and use a relatively heavy weight with a low number of repetitions.

There are a few other misconceptions about weight training worth discussing.

Will weight training leave you musclebound? If during weight training exercises you go through the full range of motion (from full extension to full contraction and back again) you'll actually become more flexible as you develop your strength and power. Becoming musclebound or limited in your flexibility or movement comes only from improper weight training methods carried to extremes.

Does weight training make you slower? Weight training has not only become part of the standard training program for most football players, but for leading sprinters as well. Valeriy Borzov, the Russian who captured the gold medals in the 100- and 200-meter dashes in the 1972 Olympics credited weight training (as part of his full training program) with helping transform him from an average sprinter to an Olympic champion. And studies have indicated that weight lifters have among the fastest reflexes of Olympic athletes.

Do muscles developed by weight lifting become flabby in later years? Many athletes, not just those who have used weights, become overweight and flabby after their sport careers end. The problem generally occurs because they continue to eat the same amount of food they did when they were actively training and competing. If you match your diet to the amount of exercise you get (which is what anyone, athlete or not, should do), you will be able to maintain both your weight and muscle tone with a minimum of conditioning and exercise.

It isn't always necessary to use a barbell in weight training. Many athletes have developed their own "overload" techniques:

—Many basketball players, including high-jumping David Thompson, have used an-

39

kle weights during practice to help increase their leaping ability.

—Uganda's John Akii Bua credited his 1972 gold medal in the Olympics 400-meter hurdles to six-day-a-week workouts of 1,500 meters over the hurdles while wearing a 25-pound weighted jacket.

—Ted Williams, like many baseball players, helped develop his wrists, arms, and shoulders by swinging a bat that had been drilled out and filled with several ounces of lead at the heavy end. Gary Player added weight to some practice golf clubs for the same reason.

However, most athletes will find using barbells and other weight equipment to be the most convenient and most efficient way to develop strength.

Most of the basic weight training exercises, including the ones given in this book, are widely used, with only slight variations from one weight training coach to another. But there is a wide difference of opinion among coaches and trainers over what training methods produce the best results.

Until recent years, there was even disagreement over how the muscle works. Now it is generally acknowledged that only a portion of the muscle fibers in any given muscle are actually contracting during most physical work. The other fibers in the muscle simply are not involved in the effort.

As the physical effort is repeated, those muscle fibers already in use begin to tire, and some of the muscle fibers that were inactive begin to contract to "pick up the slack" in the work effort. By the time the muscle is totally fatigued and unable to perform any more effort, all of the muscle fibers in that muscle have been brought into play.

This is why many modern weight training programs are based on the use of heavy weights, with the athlete doing as many repetitions as he possibly can—a technique called "working to failure."

Some coaches express concern about the greater possibility of injury with heavy weights. The Rams, for example, use lighter weights than most teams, believing that even a minimum weight training program will produce benefits, and with less risk of a player's hurting himself.

"The name of the game is availability," says Ram trainer Gary Tuthill. "All you have to do to turn a good weight program into a disaster is to hurt one key person so he can't play."

Under Tuthill's guidance, the Rams have had the most injury-free team in the NFL the last two years.

In addition to using lighter weights, the Rams'

training staff also advises the players to stay away from some of the most common weight exercises (clean and jerk, dead lift, and full squat), because these exercises carry a greater potential for injury when done with heavy weights.

Other professional teams incorporate these exercises into their weight training programs, but at least a couple of NFL players have reportedly been hurt during impromptu "weight lifting contests" during workouts.

So what type of weight training is best for you?

Most weight training experts agree that using heavy weights (that will permit only from about four to eight repetitions) will generally produce the greatest strength and size gains. Lighter weights when combined with a higher total of repetitions (10 to 15) will also produce strength gains (although not as much as heavy weights) but with less increase in muscle size.

However, Frank Egenhoff, weight training coach for the San Francisco 49ers, says that even light weights will produce size gains if the athlete "works to failure," or completes as many repetitions as he possibly can with each exercise.

If you do not want to add any more size and weight, but still want to train with weights to keep your muscle tone, Egenhoff suggests simply maintaining the same amount of weight you use in each exercise and the same number of sets and repetitions while trying to cut your workout time (for example, from a workout of 40 minutes eventually to one exactly the same that lasts only 25 minutes).

If you are a college or professional football player who needs added weight to go along with increased strength, and if your coach and trainer agree, you might consider the heavy weight approach. Still, Gary Tuthill notes that the light weight method can produce significant size gains if the player "works to failure" and follows a weight-gaining diet. Ram quarterback Ron Jaworski added 20 pounds to his 170-pound frame during a year of weight training under the Ram method, Tuthill said.

However, it is important to note that the expression "light weight method" does not mean using such light weights that you can do 20, 30, or more repetitions of the basic weight exercises. Generally speaking, you should use a weight that will allow you to do at least 6 repetitions for each exercise; when you are able to do two sets of 12 repetitions for each exercise, it is time to add weight and repeat the overloading process.

Before starting any weight training program,

there are some basic guidelines you should follow:

W A R M   U P . Suddenly lifting weights, particularly heavier weights, without a warm-up is an invitation to injury. It is a good practice to do your stretching exercises, 15 or 20 push-ups, and two minutes or so of rope skipping, before working out. Also, the first weight exercise should be a light warm-up exercise (with a light enough weight to do about 25 repetitions).

S T A R T   L I G H T . When you first begin training with weights, it is important to use only very light weights. At this stage you should concentrate on developing good form while doing the exercises. After four or five workouts you should begin to have an idea of the correct amount of weight to use for the various exercises.

G O O D   F O R M . The first repetitions of each exercise should be done very slowly as another warm-up and precaution against injury. As you begin to tire during the exercise, increase the speed of the movement (although fatigue will likely make these last repetitions as slow as the earlier ones).

Maintaining good form throughout the entire exercise is another protection against hurting yourself, while making sure that strength and flexibility are developed properly at the same time. Do as many repetitions as you can during each exercise, but when your form starts to break down, *concentrate on keeping good form so that you train and don't strain.*

A L T E R N A T E . To make the best use of your workout time, use your "rest period" after finishing one exercise to do another exercise that uses other muscles. For example, between sets of leg exercises, when the leg muscles are tired, you can still do an arm exercise as a "breather."

S C H E D U L E . Weight training should not be a daily routine. For best strength training results, a series of 7 to 10 different exercises three days a week (with at least one day of rest between workouts) is about right. However, it is a good idea to begin weight training with a workout every day for three or four days, but only with light weights in order to develop a feel for the movement and rhythm of the exercises that is essential to learning good form.

A regular workout schedule is necessary for weight training to be really effective. There's no getting around the fact that good weight training is hard work, and if you miss a workout, there is often a tendency to skip the next one as well, and so on. The best bet is to pick a time that is convenient for you (Mondays, Wednesdays, and Fridays

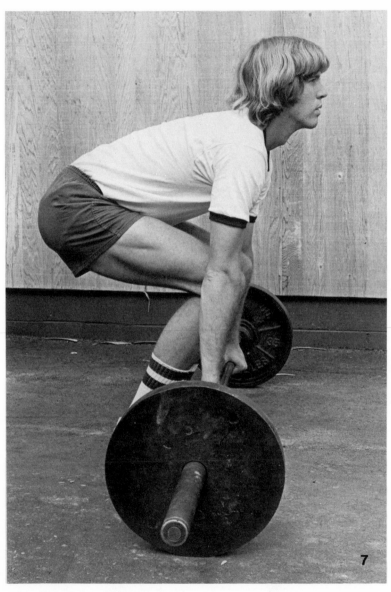

7

The dead lift is a good warm-up exercise when using a light weight. Experienced weight lifters sometimes use heavier weights in this exercise for back and leg development.

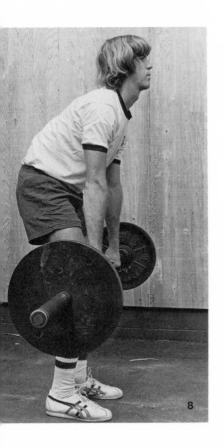

8

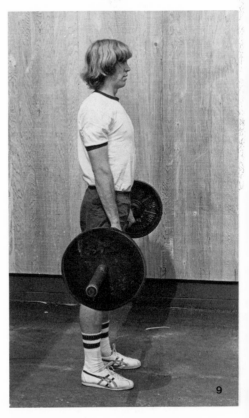

9

at noon, or after school or work, for example) and work out at those same times every week.

You should also wait about two hours after a meal before working with weights (or any other strenuous exercise, for that matter). If you find the noon hour is the best time for your weight training, you may find it more convenient to eat lunch after the workout, instead of just before it.

A cardinal rule of weight training is that, when you are first beginning to use weights, if the weight seems too heavy for you during the first repetitions, switch to a lighter weight. Using a weight that is too heavy for you, one that makes you strain and lose your form at the beginning of an exercise, can lead to an injury.

A basic, all-around program of weight training exercises is illustrated in Figs. 7–21.

1. D E A D   L I F T . As an event in power-lifting competition, the dead lift involves extremely heavy weights. Some weight training coaches also advise using heavy weights with this exercise in their programs. However, because the dead lift can lead to back problems when done with heavy weights and not executed properly, the dead lift recommended here uses light weights and is designed principally as a warm-up exercise.

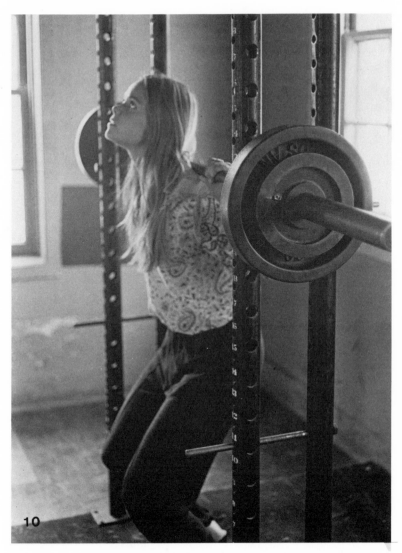

10

The squat rack allows the use of heavier weights necessary for maximum development during squat exercises. A heavy set of pins (hidden by the barbell plates) ensures that the heavy barbell will not fall if the athlete loses his balance under the heavy weight. The barbell is loaded with the weight plates while resting on these pins (which are removable and therefore can be adjusted to various heights—another set of the pins is shown in the lower part of the photo).

As a warm-up, use about one-third of your body weight and do about 15 repetitions. Gradually work up to one set of about 25 repetitions with about two-thirds of your body weight.

Technique: Stand as close to the bar as possible (this is a good practice on any lift from the ground to lessen chance of back strain during the lifting movement), feet about shoulder width apart. With hands palm down on the bar, bend at the knees and waist, keeping your back straight. Lift with both the legs and back, keeping the back straight and head up, until standing straight. Lower weight to the ground and repeat.

2. HALF-SQUAT. Considered by many weight experts to be the best single, all-around weight exercise, the half-squat is the key exercise for developing the upper leg muscles.

The half-squat is sometimes called the "parallel squat" because the top of the thighs should not be lowered below the parallel-to-ground position. The full squat, where the athlete squats as far down as possible, has long been the subject of debate among coaches and trainers. Many of them believe the full squat can result in knee damage, and the general consensus is that the possible dangers of the full squat outweigh the possible benefits.

The half-squat should be done, whenever possi-

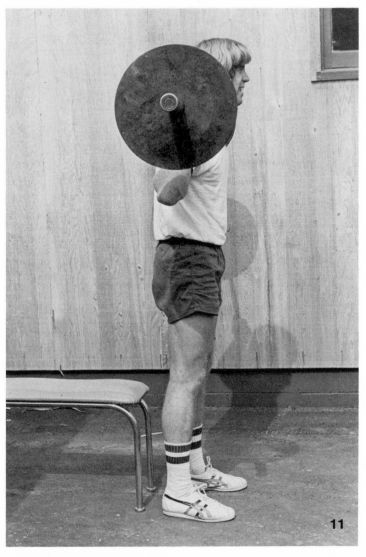

11

The half-squat is the best weight-training exercise for developing leg strength. Many weight coaches also consider it the best single weight exercise for the entire body. If a squat rack is not available, you will be limited in the exercise to the amount of weight you can lift over your head (unless you have two friends to help "spot" you and lift the weight to your back). Squatting only until your legs touch a bench or chair is a good way to keep from bending too low.

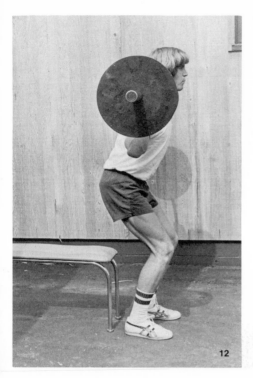

12

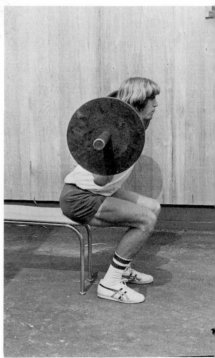

ble, in a squat rack, which allows the use of heavier weights with relative safety. If a squat rack is not available, you can use only the amount of weight you are able to lift to your shoulders—and most athletes can use considerably more weight than that eventually in the half-squat.

Technique: With your feet about shoulder width apart, back straight and head up, and weight on your shoulders, bend your legs (*keeping your back straight*) until your thighs are parallel to the ground, rise, and repeat.

Begin with about one-half to two-thirds of your weight and add weight gradually when you are able to do two sets of 12 repetitions.

3. MILITARY PRESS. Some weight coaches avoid this exercise, because the inexperienced lifter often tries to arch his back while trying to press a heavy weight, or when he tires near the end of a set of repetitions. Arching the back not only cuts down the effectiveness of the exercise as an upper body (particularly shoulder) exercise, but also can result in injury to the lower back.

However, by starting with a relatively light weight and increasing poundage gradually, the lifter will find the military press a good all-around exercise.

Technique: With feet about shoulder width

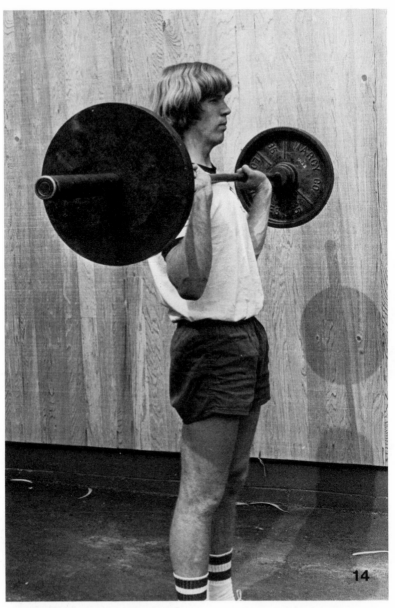

14

The military press is a good upper-body exercise. Use of a too-heavy weight too soon in this exercise, however, can lead to a possible back injury. In this and all other weight exercises, begin with light weights and gradually increase the weight as you become more experienced.

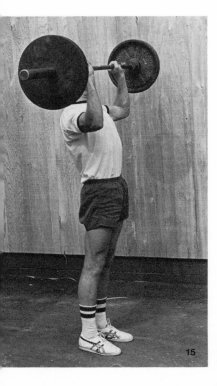

15

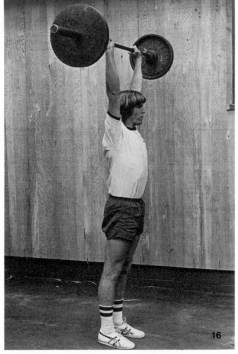

16

apart, stand close to the bar, grasp the bar palms down slightly more than shoulder width apart. Keeping your back straight, lift the bar to a rest position in front of the shoulders. Without arching your back, press the bar overhead until arms are straight. Lower to shoulder rest position and repeat.

Begin with a barbell of about one-half body weight, increasing weight gradually when you are able to do two sets of 12 repetitions.

4. BENCH PRESS. Because the lifter can use more weight with less chance of injury in the bench press than in the military press, most coaches rely on the bench press as the primary upper body exercise. Football coaches particularly emphasize this exercise for linemen, because it develops strength in the muscles (and even the basic position) used in stand-up blocking, fending off blocking, and other line play.

Technique: Keeping your back flat on the bench, with your hands slightly wider than shoulder width apart, lower the bar until it touches your shoulder, and then press it up until arms are straight. Repeat. (In the bench press and other weight exercises, the muscles benefit from the *lowering* phase of the exercise, as well as the *press* movement. Proper breathing is also important: in-

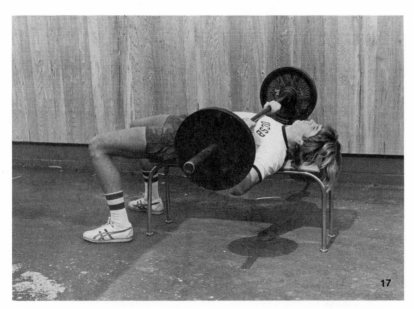

The bench press is the one exercise used by nearly every athlete in weight training, whatever his or her sport, because it is perhaps the best all-around upper-body weight exercise and can be done with relatively little chance of injury. This is another exercise that requires a rack to hold the weight while the athlete positions himself on the bench, or requires a "spotter"—a friend who can assist in giving the weights to the one exercising and taking them from him when he has completed the exercise.

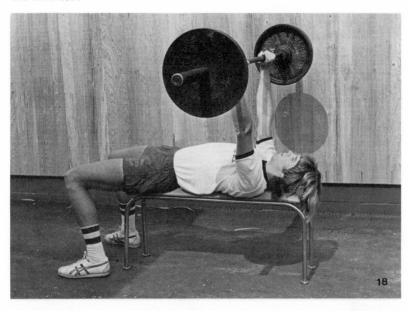

hale during the lowering phase, and exhale during the press or exertion phase. This same breathing pattern should be followed in all weight exercises.)

Begin with one-half to two-thirds of your body weight, and add weight when you are able to do two sets of 12 repetitions.

5. S I T - U P S . One bent leg sit-up is worth about ten sit-ups done either with the legs straight or with the feet held down, according to UCLA's Jim Bush. When the legs are bent during the sit-up, the abdominal muscles are forced to do the major effort in the exercise.

Weak abdominals are a major cause of back pains (see Chapter 6), and because the abdominals assist other muscle groups during a wide variety of athletic movements, conditioning them is essential for athletic fitness.

Technique: With knees bent and feet kept on the floor, *roll* up (rather than "jerk" up) until your forehead goes between your knees. Do as many as you can, working up to 50. Some athletes, to make the effort more difficult, hold a weight plate (usually 5 or 10 pounds) behind their head during the exercise.

There are other weight exercises that, depending on your sport, you may want to incorporate into a training program (see Chapter 6). These

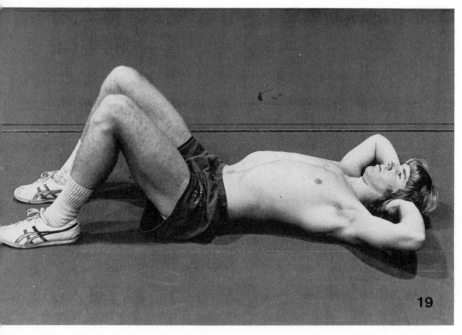

19

The sit-up is usually done without weights, although many athletes hold a weight plate behind their head during the exercise. The bent leg sit-up, shown here, is a much better exercise than sit-ups done either with the legs straight or with the feet held down by a friend. (PHOTOS: PONCE)

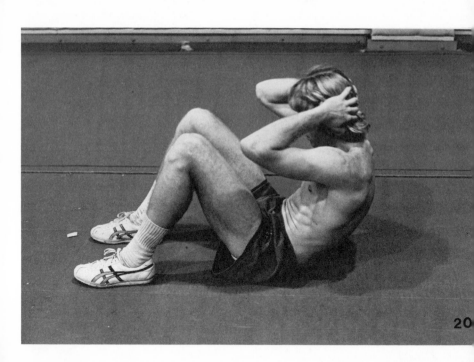

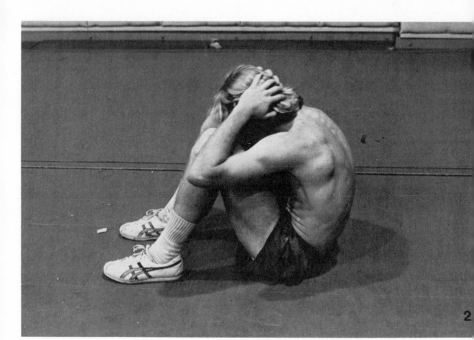

include swinging a weighted bat (baseball) or club (golf), or running up stadium steps while wearing a weighted belt—an exercise used by athletes in many sports, including football, basketball, volleyball, and track, where muscular endurance and strength in the legs are important.

If your sport involves jumping—such as basketball, volleyball, or the high jump—you should consider including the *depth jump* in your training schedule.

Used by several world-class high jumpers in recent years, including recent world holder Pat Matzdorf, the depth jump is an exhausting exercise for the legs that should be saved until the end of a weight-training workout. Coaches have theorized that the depth jump improves jumping ability by conditioning the "reactive ability" of the leg muscles and nerves, enabling the athlete to speed up the leg extension movement in the jump. Placekicker Jan Stenerud has said the depth jumps which he started while training for ski jumping also helped his leg strength for kicking.

Technique: Simply jump from a table (about 36 inches in height) onto a soft gym mat, and as soon as you land, jump up as high as you can. The faster you can jump after landing, the more you will benefit from it. (Jumping onto a hard surface is likely to cause knee problems.) Repeat 25 times.

In recent years, many professional teams have included the use of various weight training machines and devices, along with "free" weights (barbells and dumbbells) in their training programs.

The most familiar of these machines are the Nautilus and the Universal Gym. Each has its supporters among coaches and athletes.

Manufacturers of both claim that their machines are superior to barbells because they work on the principle of "variable resistance." Essentially, this theory is based on the fact that in any given exercise (such as the military or bench press), the athlete is able to lift more weight during most of the movement than he is right at the beginning of the movement, when his leverage is poorest.

Because the machines are geared so that the athlete is always exerting his full potential throughout the entire range of movement (during the last repetitions of a set in particular), the manufacturers claim, the athlete utilizes his maximum ability while working to failure.

The machines are expensive, but have won converts: The 49ers have switched to the Nautilus machines exclusively for their weight training. The Rams currently use both the Nautilus and the Universal Gym, as well as barbell equipment. Gary Tuthill says that one reason the Rams continue to use free weights (barbells and dumbbells) is that football is a game of coordination and balance, and working with free weights helps develop both of these

Most of the exercises on the weight machines are similar to those done with free weights, and the basic training methods (warm up, start light, good form, etc.) are the same as for exercises with barbells.

Another machine now being used by a few professional teams is the Cybex. Although the machine is primarily designed for rehabilitation, it has other capabilities. The 49ers use their Cybex not only as an exerciser for injured players but also as a testing device.

On both gauges and printed graph readouts, the Cybex measures strength and power of key muscle groups. The 49ers use this information in a number of ways.

For example, if a 49er has had knee surgery in the off season, the trainer can record and compare the output of the muscles of both legs. If the quadriceps (thigh) group of the leg that had the sur-

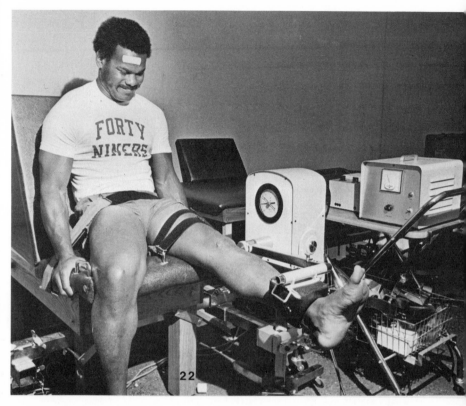

Edgar Hardy, a San Francisco 49ers lineman, demonstrates the leg raise as he exercises on a Cybex machine following knee surgery in the off season. (PHOTO: MALDONADO)

gery shows only 55 percent of the strength of the other leg, it will be obvious to the trainer—and the athlete—that more conditioning is needed for the recuperating leg. (Sometimes the machine has good news. When Willie Harper, 49er linebacker, arrived in training camp after off-season knee surgery, the Cybex showed that his "bad" leg was actually 15 percent stronger than his normal, healthy leg—evidence to the trainer of the effort Harper had put into exercising the leg after the operation.)

The Cybex has also been used to predict injury. Experience has shown that muscle pulls in the upper leg are likely for players if hamstrings are not about 60 to 70 percent as strong as the quadriceps, according to the 49er staff. When a Cybex test shows a ratio much different from that, the trainers can design a weight training program that will correct the imbalance and thereby hope to prevent an injury.

In addition to machines such as the Nautilus, Universal Gym, and Cybex (which may cost anywhere from $2,000 to $5,000 or more), there is also a host of rope and pulley gadgets and devices (Exer-Genie, Powerex) on the market. Most are relatively inexpensive (beginning at about $15), light, and compact, making them easy to take

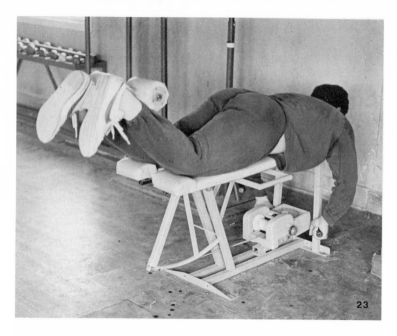

One of several "accommodating resistance" weight-training devices, the Mini-Gym unit shown here has been set up for use with an exercise primarily aimed at developing the hamstring muscles at the back of the upper leg.

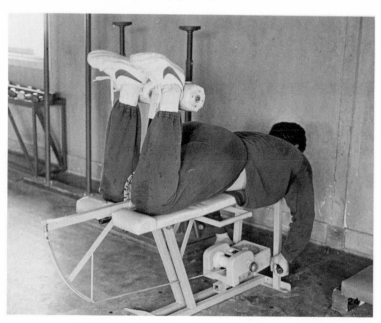

along on a vacation. For the occasional athlete, and especially for those who either dislike weight training or don't have access to weights, these devices may help develop strength and maintain muscle tone. Some professional teams have also included some of these devices in their conditioning programs. Jeff Snedecker, New York Jets trainer, credited one of the devices, the Mini-Gym, with helping Joe Namath recover from one of his knee operations.

4. Flexibility

WHEN THE Oakland A's tightly muscled power hitter Reggie Jackson was plagued by a pulled hamstring muscle prior to the World Series in 1974, he told reporters that he was going to begin stretching exercises in the off season in an attempt to ease the problem.

Several trainers say that if Jackson had been doing the stretching exercises for the preceding two years, he probably never would have had the muscle pulls in the first place—or at least they might have been only minor pulls.

Stretching exercises are not new. Track coaches have been having their athletes do them for years.

But in the last couple of years, stretching exercises have become incorporated in the conditioning

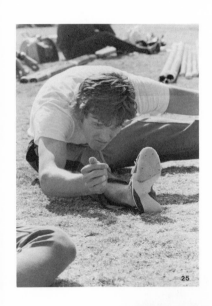

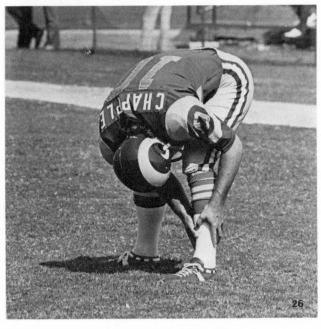

Bob Seagren, world-record pole vaulter and also a top finisher in the Superstars competition, and Dave Chapple, former NFL punting leader with the L.A. Rams, are shown warming up with two stretching exercises designed to stretch leg and back muscles. (PHOTOS: PONCE)

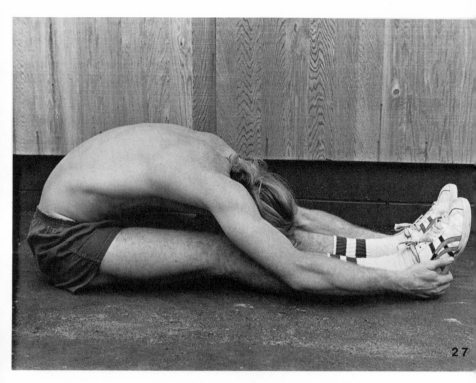

The sit reach is probably the most important single stretching exercise for most athletes because it will stretch the muscles of the lower back as well as the muscles along the back of the leg—primarily the hamstrings—that are so vulnerable to muscle pulls. Don't be surprised if you are unable either to reach your feet or to bend your head between your knees (as shown here by Gus Mee) when you first begin stretching. It takes most athletes several months of slow but steady stretching before they become this flexible. Keep legs straight, knees locked during exercise.

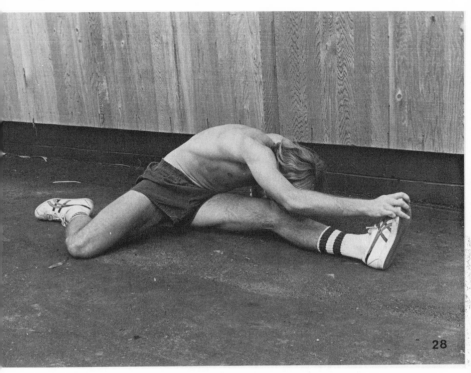

28

Another favorite flexibility exercise for the back and leg muscles is the hurdler's stretch. As with the sit reach (and all other stretching exercises), stretch only to the point of tightness and then hold that position for about five seconds. Trying to stretch too quickly or straining to reach too far is likely to defeat the purpose of the exercise by causing a muscle strain. Keep leg straight during exercise.

programs of teams in nearly every major sport, from football and baseball to hockey and swimming.

Why stretch?

Stretching exercises do not build strength or endurance, but because they are one of the best guarantees against a wide range of injuries—particularly hamstring and groin pulls—for the professional athlete or any serious athlete they can be just as important as running or weight training exercises.

Muscle pulls, a common occurrence at training camps in a lot of sports, can largely be prevented if the athletes maintain a year-round flexibility program. Professional football teams learned this the hard way last year when one result of the players' strike was a rash of muscle pulls among the players who had failed to stretch in the off season and were trying to get in shape in a hurry.

Players have also found that off-season stretching eliminates much of the stiffness and pain that accompanies the early part of training camp. Also, any stiffness that does occur can be eased with stretching exercises before and after a workout.

Stretching programs have become so popular that several teams, including the San Francisco 49ers and the Los Angeles Rams, have completely

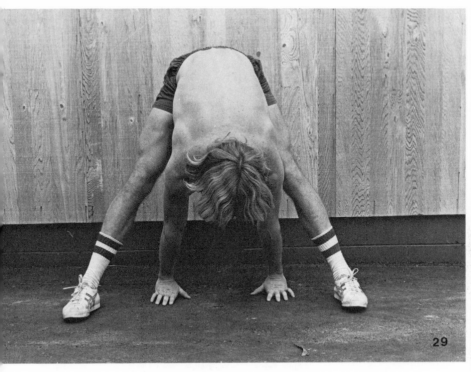

The groin stretcher will increase flexibility in the muscles on the inside of the upper leg, as well as other leg and back muscles. Again, this exercise should not be done quickly (it is not a bouncing toe-toucher) but should be done slowly, held five seconds, and then repeated.

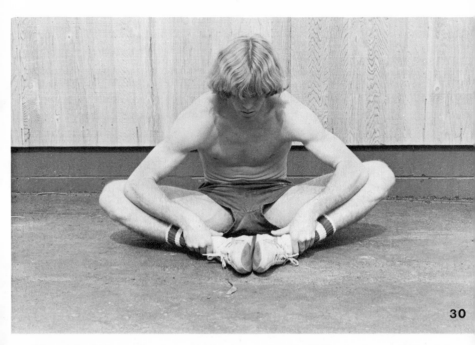

The groin sit is another exercise for increasing flexibility in the muscles of the groin area. Gently try to push your knees down to the ground.

replaced traditional calisthenics (which Ram trainer Gary Tuthill describes as the "herky-jerky toe touchers and jumping jacks") with stretching exercises.

Tuthill credits the program in part for the fact that over the last two years the Rams have had the most injury-free record in the NFL.

Los Angeles Dodger trainer Bill Buhler said the stretching exercises Steve Garvey had been doing helped him stay in the lineup when he was injured in 1974, on the way to a season that ended with Garvey's being named the National League's most valuable player.

An athlete who has been doing a lot of running to get in shape especially needs to include stretching exercises in his daily routine. Running tends to develop but also to tighten the muscles at the back of the leg, including the hamstring and calf muscles. In turn, as these muscles tighten, the Achilles tendon becomes shorter.

Runners occasionally have problems with Achilles tendinitis, which can result in severe pain at the heel or where the tendon joins the calf muscle. This commonly occurs when the Achilles tendon, which tends to be somewhat inflexible, is strained.

Exercises that stretch the back of the leg and the

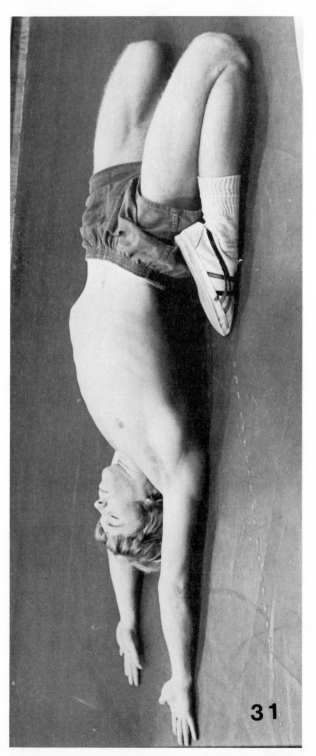

The quad stretch is designed to stretch the quadriceps muscles in the front of the upper legs. From a sitting position (sitting between your feet), slowly lean back and try to touch your head and back to the floor. A variation of this exercise can be done during the hurdler's stretch: With one leg straight in front of you and the other bent back (see Fig. 28), lean backward, again trying to touch head and back to the floor.

31

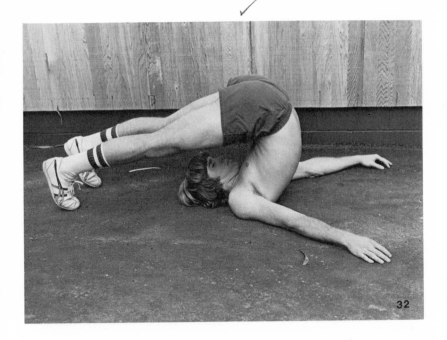

The shoulder stand will increase flexibility in the upper back, hamstrings, and groin. Keep knees locked during exercise and try to touch feet to the ground. Caution: This exercise should not be attempted if you are suffering from low back pains.

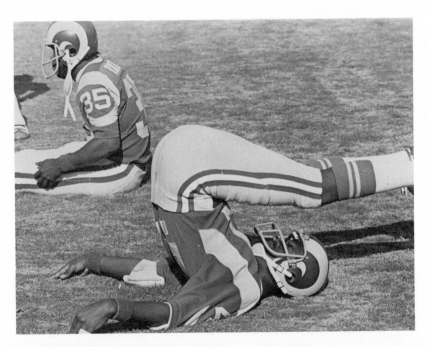

Achilles tendon not only reduce the chance of Achilles tendinitis, but also lessen the risk of one of the most feared injuries in sports—a rupture of the Achilles tendon, which can occur if Achilles tendinitis is not treated.

As an athlete gets older, flexibility becomes even more important.

Range of motion tends to decrease with age and recovering from an injury takes longer, which means that getting back into shape after an injury also takes longer. Sometimes the result is a career brought to a premature end, such as when basketball great Jerry West decided to retire after muscle pulls had hampered his play during his last years with the Los Angeles Lakers.

One of the best things about stretching exercises is that they make it possible to achieve an adequate level of flexibility in very little time. Two or three minutes a day is usually enough for anyone except the professional or fulltime athlete, who should spend up to 10 to 20 minutes a day stretching.

To be effective, stretching should be done year round.

However, don't expect overnight results. If you are starting a stretching routine in the off season, don't worry if you seem very tight. What is important is how flexible you are at the start of the season.

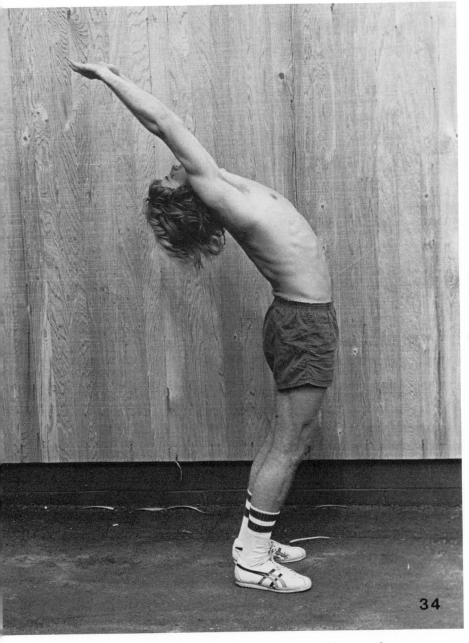

34

The sun reach helps loosen both back and shoulder muscles.

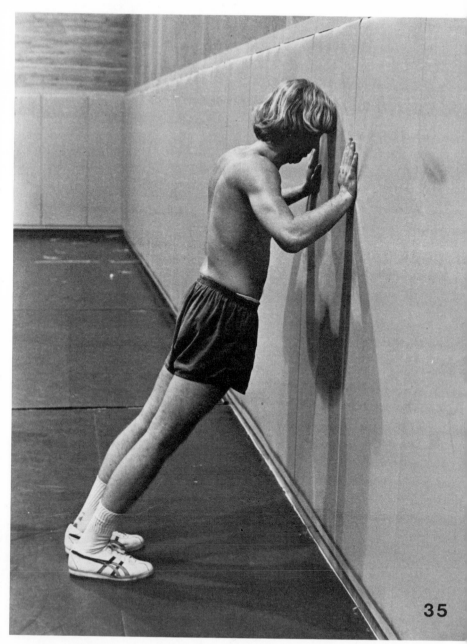

35

The wall dip is a key exercise for stretching the Achilles tendon. Simply stand a few feet away from a wall and, keeping your legs straight and feet flat on the ground, lean slowly toward the wall as shown.

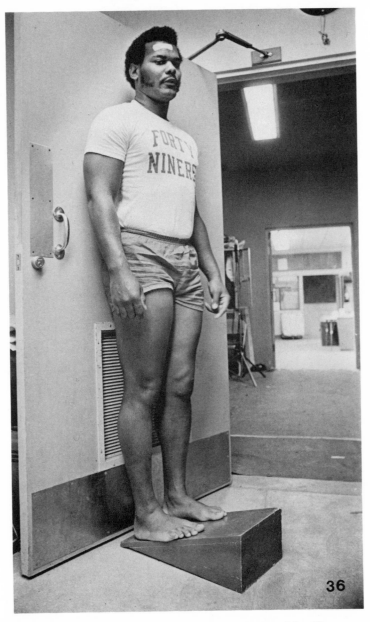

36

Edgar Hardy of the 49ers stands on a box designed by 49ers trainer Chuck Krpata to help stretch the Achilles tendon and muscles along the back of the leg. Players who have had problems with hamstring pulls or tightness at the back of the heel will stand on this box for up to about 10 minutes before a practice or game. (PHOTO: MALDONADO)

DON'T STRAIN. Stretch *slowly* to your *comfortable* limit. *Don't cheat* (by bending a leg that is supposed to be kept straight), but when you reach the point where the stretch starts to become uncomfortable, you should always stop. After you become more accustomed to stretching, you'll find that when you reach your limit, and relax and hold that position, you can then take up a little slack by stretching just slightly more.

REPEAT. Each exercise should be repeated at least twice, and preferably three or four times. Each time try to stretch just a bit further, but again, not to the point where it becomes uncomfortable.

DON'T BOUNCE. An important part of the stretching program to remember is not to "bounce" in an effort. The most common injury that occurs during stretching happens when someone reaches down to touch his toes, finds he can't quite do it, and so bounces down in an effort to reach them, and in doing so, strains a muscle along the back of his leg. Instead, do each exercise *slowly* and stretch only to the point of tightness.

5. Athletic Diet

Russian gymnast Olga Korbut will put ketchup on almost any food, tennis star Chris Evert snacks on honey between matches, golfer Al Geiberger packed peanut butter and jelly sandwiches around with him on the way to a PGA championship, and basketball's Bill Walton is a vegetarian.

So, what is the best diet for an athlete?

That question is usually left up to the individual athlete to answer. The San Francisco 49ers, like most professional sport teams, provide meals with a balanced variety of foods, but except in special cases (an overweight player, or one who is on a diet prescribed by a doctor) the actual choice of foods at each meal is made by the players themselves.

"By the time a player has played football this long, he generally knows what will agree with him, and what he can play best on," says Chuck Krpata, 49er trainer.

UCLA's Jim Bush adds that he has seen runners eat the worst possible "junk food" dinner one night and come back the next day to set a world record.

Nevertheless, just as most other sports have followed the lead of track and swimming in endurance training and flexibility exercises, more and more athletes, coaches, and trainers from all areas in athletics are beginning to learn what runners and swimmers have discovered in recent years—diet, like conditioning, can be a factor in performance and should be a matter of year-round concern.

There is a good reason why track and swimming have been at the forefront of dietary activity in athletics: Performances in both sports can be measured with a stop watch and tape measure. A runner, for example, who changes his diet can see the evidence of the change in his clockings over a period of time. In most other sports there is no such clearcut way to gauge performance.

Of course, dietary requirements vary among

sports. Size and weight may be advantageous to the football player, but not to the long distance runner; and the athlete who is in training will have considerably different nutritional needs than the weekend golfer.

But whatever his sport, the athlete should realize that complete, maximum conditioning depends in part on a good diet, and also that a bad diet can actually hurt his ability to perform at peak capabilities.

WEIGHT CONTROL

Most athletes never give a second thought to diet unless they are trying either to lose weight or to gain it.

Losing weight is the most common concern.

There are very few athletes who are both fat and quick. Those few would be even quicker with less weight, and because most sports place a premium on quickness, the fat athlete is likely always to be the exception rather than the rule.

Consequently, the first thing about an athlete a coach usually checks is his weight.

In professional sports, sometimes the best athletes show up in training camp overweight after an off season of lecturing on the "banquet circuit" and eating oversized, fattening meals day after day with few opportunities for regular exercise. Quite a few World Series heroes have blamed the banquet trail for their poor showing the following year.

While a professional team may put up with a top athlete who arrives in camp with extra poundage, most teams won't waste the time it takes for an overweight rookie or average player to get into shape.

Coaches know that the time spent trying to lose weight in training is time that could have been used to reach peak athletic fitness if the athlete had been in good shape from the start.

Most important, the body of an overweight athlete simply cannot operate as efficiently as one without extra, unnecessary pounds. *The overweight body will begin to fatigue earlier—and fatigue leads to both a drop-off in performance and an increased likelihood of injury.*

What is your best or "ideal" weight?

It is the weight at which you perform best, have the greatest endurance and strength for your particular sport.

Most charts showing ideal weights for men and women are somewhat misleading for athletes. If you are a distance runner, for example, your best weight for running may be 10 to 20 percent below the ideal weight generally recommended for a person of your build. On the other hand, the football player who has trained with weights may be 30 to 40 pounds over a suggested ideal weight and still not be overweight, if the extra weight is largely thick bone structure and heavy muscle mass rather than fat.

In recent years, a few professional teams have followed the lead of the San Francisco 49ers in measuring the fat and lean content of the players' body weight in an effort to determine their best playing weight.

However, the fat–lean test conducted by these teams requires certain equipment and access to a water tank or swimming pool because part of the test involves weighing the athlete in water.

The "pinch test" is a simple method anyone can use to determine his or her appropriate fat content.

With your thumb and forefinger (or better yet, a set of calipers), pinch the fold of skin at your triceps, the muscle at the back of the upper arm between the elbow and shoulder. For the athlete, the pinched fold between the two fingers should measure about one-half inch or less. If the fold measures more than about one inch, your fat content is too high, even if your weight seems to be about normal.

If you are overweight (or have too much fat content) it is basically (barring medical problems) because your intake of calories while eating has been greater than your expenditure of calories during exercise and other daily activities.

The food you eat is the "fuel" for the body. A *calorie* (actually a unit of heat in physics) is the common measure of heat or "energy" yielded by different foods. If you take in more calories of fuel than you can use, that extra fuel is stored in the body as fat, which can be converted back to fuel if the body's normal fuel supply runs short.

However, most people (and even many athletes) seldom exert themselves to the point where their normal fuel supplies become depleted. Consequently their fat supplies simply remain as fat, and perhaps increase.

The key to weight control is simple: Match the amount of fuel you take in with the amount of fuel you burn up or use. If you take in more fuel than you burn up, you will gain weight; if you burn up more fuel than you take in, you will lose weight.

However, you should not expect overnight results.

Weight control—like endurance, strength, and flexibility conditioning—takes time and effort.

Each year, newly developed "fast working" diets become popular. For most individuals, but *particularly for athletes*, these "fad" diets not only are inadequate but can actually be dangerous.

The athlete, especially the athlete in training, needs a well-balanced diet in order to be supplied with essential minerals and vitamins, as well as the other basic food elements. Studies have shown that minerals, in particular, play a crucial role in athletic performance, and the latest "grapefruit" diet —or "zen" diet or "high fat" diet—probably will not meet the nutritional demands of your sport.

What should the athletic diet include?

Basically, there are two types of food used by the body for fuel (carbohydrates and fats), one used mainly for growth and repair of the body (proteins), and three components needed by the body to control and regulate its functions (minerals, vitamins, and water).

CARBOHYDRATES: The sugars and starches—carbohydrates—are the major energy source for the athlete. Because carbohydrates require less oxygen than fats to be converted into fuel, they are the primary source of energy during short-term physical exertion. *Best sources:* cereals and grains (wheat, rice, corn, and oats) and the foods made from them (spaghetti, macaroni, and bread), potatoes, dry beans, soybeans, nuts, and the natural sugars in fruits.

F A T S : Fats are actually a more concentrated source of energy than carbohydrates, and because only limited amounts of carbohydrates can be stored in the body, fats take over as the major fuel source as the supply of carbohydrates is depleted in long-term endurance exercise. *Best sources:* meats, vegetable oils, dairy products, and nuts.

P R O T E I N S : Not a major energy source for the athlete, proteins are essential for building muscle tissue and general body growth, and (as enzymes) control the body's reactions and processes. *Best sources:* meat, fish, dairy products, eggs, soybeans, and beans.

M I N E R A L S A N D V I T A M I N S : Not a direct source of energy in themselves, minerals and vitamins act as regulators in the functioning of the body's systems, growth, and utilization of energy. For the athlete, the most important minerals are calcium, iron, magnesium, phosphorus, potassium, and sodium, while the essential vitamins include the A, B-complex, C, D, and E vitamins. Minerals and vitamins occur in a wide variety of foods, and a well-balanced diet will provide the amounts necessary for basic health requirements. In endurance athletic competition mineral loss can be severe and some minerals should be replaced during or just after the activity.

W A T E R : Another regulator in the body, water is taken in daily by the body not only in liquids, but also in food, such as fruits and vegetables, many of which may contain more than 90 percent water. Water loss during athletic activity can be serious, even critical.

The best athletic diets include all of these major elements.

The simplest way to guarantee that your daily food intake is meeting basic nutritional requirements is to follow the "Essential Four" plan based on the Recommended Daily Dietary Allowances developed by the Food and Nutrition Board of the National Academy of Sciences.

This plan categorizes foods into four groups (meat, vegetable–fruit, milk products, and bread–cereal), and recommends at least two to four servings from each group each day:

M E A T   G R O U P (*two or more of the following servings per day*): Two to three ounces of lean, cooked meat, poultry, or fish; two eggs; one cup of cooked dry beans, dry peas, or lentils; four tablespoons of peanut butter. (For example, it would be possible to meet the daily recommendation for the meat group with a three-ounce serving of chicken *and* one egg *and* one-half cup of cooked dry peas; or by eating two cups of cooked dry beans.)

V E G E T A B L E – F R U I T   G R O U P   (*four or more of the following servings per day*): One-half cup of vegetable or fruit, or ordinary portion (whole apple, orange, banana, or half cantaloupe or grapefruit). Although all fruits and vegetables are basically interchangeable in this group, it is recommended for athletes that of the four daily servings, at least one serving be a citrus fruit (for Vitamin C) and another serving be either a dark green or deep yellow vegetable (for Vitamin A).

M I L K   P R O D U C T S   G R O U P   (*two or more of the following servings per day*): Eight ounces (one cup) of milk. (The following may be substituted for four ounces or one-half cup of milk: one-inch cube of cheddar or other hard cheese; one-half cup of yogurt; three-fourths cup of cottage cheese; three-fourths cup of ice cream.) Although the plan recommends at least two servings per day for adults, it suggests teen-agers should have at least four servings per day.

B R E A D – C E R E A L   G R O U P   (*four or more of the following servings per day*): One slice of bread; one ounce ready-to-eat cereal, three-fourths cup of cooked cereal, spaghetti, rice, grits, or noodles.

There is no such thing as a "perfect" athletic diet, but the Essential Four plan does provide the good, solid nutritional foundation for a diet for athletes.

And the plan is also a safe but effective diet for an athlete who wants to lose weight.

For the average person, eating only the minimum recommendations in the Essential Four plan (two servings each of meat and milk products, and four servings each from the fruit–vegetable and bread–cereal groups daily) will provide approximately 50 to 75 percent of the daily calories needed to maintain his or her weight.

The plan assumes that other foods such as fats, sugar and other sweets, syrups, oils are generally included in the average diet, and therefore help fill out the daily caloric requirements *after* ensuring that the essential foods have provided basic nutritional needs.

However, the athlete who is trying to lose weight can skip the unnecessary (and generally fattening) foods, and *meet his daily nutritional needs while losing weight* by sticking to the minimum recommendations of the Essential Four groups.

If those minimum recommendations still leave you hungry (if, for example, you are trying to lose weight and training hard at the same time), most

93

authorities agree you can eat additional servings from the fruit–vegetable group each day without gaining unwanted pounds.

Exercise itself, of course, plays a key role in any attempt to lose weight.

Studies at Harvard indicate that if your caloric intake remains the same, you can expect to lose between 16 and 26 pounds in one year by including a half hour of moderate exercise in your daily routine.

If the exercise is more vigorous, such as swimming or running, you can lose about two pounds a week by exercising for about an hour a day while maintaining your normal diet.

One additional benefit of vigorous exercise, the type an athlete in training should be getting, is that the body continues to burn fuel or calories at an above-normal rate for some time (up to several hours) after strenuous exercise.

The most effective approach to losing weight combines exercise with a cutback in calorie intake. The main advantage of following the Essential Four plan outlined above (along with the fact that it supplies basic nutritional needs) is that it does away with the need to count calories, which can be confusing and time-consuming. Another way to achieve similar results (assuming you already eat a well-balanced diet) is to cut down the size of your food servings or portions.

In either case, if you are trying to lose weight you should *avoid* eating the following:

Beer, wine, liquor
Cakes, pies, pastries
Candy, chocolate
Potato chips, pretzels, similar snack foods
Gravies, sauces

Some athletes are concerned not about losing weight, but about gaining it.

But it does little good just to add pounds in the way of fat. Most weight-gaining programs developed for football players include weight training (barbell or weight machine) exercises as well as a special diet to ensure that the weight gained by a player shows up as increased muscle size rather than as a spare tire around his middle.

Without weight training, it is unlikely that an athlete can gain a significant amount of useful (muscle tissue, not fat) weight after he has passed his growing years, up to nineteen or twenty.

However, any weight-gaining diet should not include just milkshakes and other high calorie foods, but instead should have a well-balanced diet—such as the Essential Four plan—as its base.

High school athletes and others up to about twenty years of age require more protein during their years of growth and development.

Professional teams usually give players trying to gain weight powdered protein and carbohydrate supplements, and tell them to eat more foods high in these two elements during meals—but for different reasons. The carbohydrates are an energy source, and additional carbohydrates in a diet are insurance against depleting energy reserves to the point where fats begin to be used to supply energy for the body. Proteins, on the other hand, are given for their role in the growth of muscle tissue.

However, some studies have indicated that excessive amounts of protein in a diet are largely wasted, because the body cannot use overly great amounts of protein for tissue building and repair purposes. It is likely that high school athletes, or athletes attempting to gain weight, will benefit only from up to one gram of protein per day for each two pounds of body weight. For example, the 180-pound athlete can effectively use only about 90 grams of protein. (An eight-ounce glass of milk contains about 9 grams of protein, an egg about 6 grams, two slices of bacon about 5 grams, three ounces of beef about 22 to 25.)

If you are trying to gain weight, instead of eating three huge meals each day, it's better to eat four or more meals throughout the day to allow for better digestion.

But if you eat between meals, it is important that when you snack, you eat good, nutritious food (whole grain bread, nuts, fruit, beans) rather than "junk" or common snack foods that have little in the way of nutritional value.

DIET AND PERFORMANCE

"Carbohydrate loading" is a growing trend among many athletes who have turned to diet studies in an effort to find some slight edge in performance.

Developed originally in Europe, carbohydrate loading is based on tests that show a diet high in carbohydrates in the days just before a competition can boost an athlete's endurance dramatically.

The primary source of energy for short-term exercise (probably no more than two to four hours) is *glycogen,* a starch that the body converts from carbohydrates and stores in both the liver and muscles. It is the muscular glycogen that is most important to the athlete, because the amount of glycogen stored in an athlete's muscle tissue will in large part determine how long those muscles will be able to function before exhaustion—not just fatigue—sets in.

Unfortunately, the body is able to store only relatively small amounts of glycogen in the muscles, although tests have shown athletes who develop their endurance conditioning extensively are able to store more of it than others. The increase, not surprisingly, shows up in the athlete's best conditioned muscles—runners, for example, have their highest levels of muscular glycogen in the leg muscles.

Glycogen begins to play an important role in an athlete's performance in endurance events that stretch over several hours—such as distance running or swimming, long bicycle races, cross-country skiing, or a day-long or two-day tournament in tennis, handball, or beach volleyball.

Of course, eventually the body's store of glycogen is depleted in a sustained endurance activity. Recent research indicates that muscle tissues are able to store only enough glycogen to last about two hours, or about 20 miles when running. After that, such as in a 26-mile marathon race, the muscles have to rely on energy stored in fat. However, as John Brennand, a veteran marathon runner notes, only a well-conditioned athlete is able to compete on fat energy; by the time fat energy comes into play, the not-in-top-shape athlete is probably hurting too much to go on much longer.

The carbohydrate loading plan goes like this: About seven days before your competition, go through a workout about as long and hard as the actual competition approaching in a week, in order to deplete your stores of muscular glycogen. During the next three days eat as little carbohydrate as possible, and instead try to eat just protein and fat (meats, poultry, fish, dairy products, eggs), as well as green beans, lettuce, and celery, while continuing your normal training workouts.

In the final three days before the competition, resume your normal, balanced diet, but increase the number of carbohydrates, particularly at snack times. These additional carbohydrates could include whole grain breads and cereals, pastries, ice cream and nuts, in addition to meals featuring spaghetti, noodles, potatoes, or dried beans. It is important not to overeat or stuff yourself, but rather just to eat a higher percentage of carbohydrates during the final three days, when most athletes normally begin to taper off their training workouts.

Does it work?

Some tests have shown that carbohydrate loading apparently allowed test subjects to perform exercise (on a treadmill or stationary bicycle) up to twice as long as with their normal, balanced diets.

In actual competition it may be another story. UCLA's Jim Bush thinks any "lift" an athlete feels from the diet is largely psychological. "If you are 'up,' you are ready," he says.

Bush, who admits that he's "slow to jump on any bandwagon for something that is supposed to bring success when I've been having success," also notes that some studies have recently indicated that carbohydrate loading appears to have a "shock" effect on some individuals that may do more harm than good. Because the theory of carbohydrate loading is relatively new and the effects uncertain, many authorities recommend using the loading technique only on an infrequent basis—say, a couple of times a year at most.

Bush also suggests that it is quite common for runners unconsciously to follow a type of carbohydrate loading diet in the week before a track meet, eating lots of meat early in the week, and more snacks, junk food, and foods high in carbohydrates late in the week.

Although he lets his track athletes eat what they want on the night before a Saturday meet, Bush does tell them that it is that Friday night meal they perform on. He himself recommends a "fairly heavy meal," including steak and potatoes for the night before competition. He also suggests avoiding any greasy foods the day of competition because they are harder to digest.

Another concern in endurance competition is water and mineral loss—particularly in hot weather.

San Francisco 49er trainer Chuck Krpata says some of the football players on the squad have lost up to 28 pounds during a game! But by regulating fluid and mineral intake, problems due to heat have been kept to a minimum, he says.

Krpata's most vivid memory of what heat can do to a football team occurred at Miami in 1973, where on the artificial turf playing field temperatures reached 125 degrees during the game. Expecting the worse, Krpata had given the 49er players increased mineral (particularly potassium) supplies and more fluids for four to five days prior to the game. During the game, iced towels were kept available, and at halftime players were stripped and mopped with cool towels. Despite the precautions, the 49ers still lost five players to heat exhaustion during that game.

Recent studies have shown that it is loss of

fluids, rather than loss of salts, that causes most heat-related problems for athletes.

Yet many football coaches, who teach the way they themselves were taught, refuse to allow water for players during practices. Los Angeles Ram trainer Gary Tuthill says coaches are "crazy not to have water breaks," especially during hot weather.

The Rams, like many top professional teams, provide players with both iced water and iced Gatorade during practices as well as games.

If a game is played on a hot day, Tuthill says, "we try to get as much water as we can in the players during the first half." The reason, he says, is that if you wait until an athlete is thirsty to give him fluids, he's already lost more fluids than can be replaced during the game itself.

Salt tablets, once dispensed freely to athletes, are now given a bit more cautiously. Citing studies at Ohio State, Tuthill recommends an athlete's taking one potassium–sodium chloride combination tablet for each six pounds of weight loss during exercise. "Other than that, water is sufficient," he says.

Bush, who also agrees that it is not the lack of salt but the lack of water that causes most heat stress, nonetheless gives his runners about four salt tablets a day—always with meals—during training. They usually take two with breakfast, and one each with lunch and dinner. (Top motorcyclist Gene Romero said he favors a heavily salted steak after a hot day in racing leathers.)

What is important, Bush maintains, is to keep the body's salt in balance at all times.

Some athletes favor low salt diets, believing that if the body gets used to low salt requirements, then it takes less salt replacement to keep the body's systems in balance.

Many fruits and vegetables contain natural minerals, and it is quite possible to obtain all the necessary minerals, including salt, for normal day-to-day living just by eating a well-balanced diet—and avoiding the salt shaker both in cooking and at the table.

After becoming acclimated to a low salt intake (best accomplished during cool weather months), athletes, especially some distance runners, have found they can perform better in hot weather competition. Volleyball players who had been plagued with a salty sweat that stung their eyes and hampered their play during weekend summer beach tournaments found that after eliminating cooking and table salt from their diet they sweated less, and the perspiration that did work into their eyes did not sting.

Because an athlete's water and minerals are depleted during exercise, particularly on hot or humid days, many teams use Gatorade or similar "exercise fluids" developed in recent years.

For an athlete, the minerals that seem to most affect performance when depleted during exercise are sodium, chlorine, potassium, magnesium, and calcium. By increasing his supplies of these fluid electrolytes (*and water*) before competition in hot weather (and replacing them during competition, when possible, and immediately afterward), the athlete can largely avoid such heat stress symptoms as early fatigue, muscle cramps, or heat exhaustion.

S O D I U M : Sodium and chlorine are usually supplied together, perhaps excessively, as table salt —sodium chloride. Sodium is also present in such foods as pretzels, salted nuts, cold sandwich meats, and many "convenience" foods, such as TV dinners. It also occurs naturally in nearly all vegetables, such fruits as strawberries and apples, and kelp or seaweed.

C H L O R I N E : In addition to sodium chloride, sources of chlorine include leafy green vegetables, milk, and meat.

P O T A S S I U M : Studies indicate that the need for potassium, a key regulator in the functioning of muscles, increases as salt intake increases. Sources include all vegetables (particularly beets, tomatoes, turnips, and beans), fruits (including dried fruits), nuts, and whole, unrefined grains.

M A G N E S I U M : Best sources are leafy green vegetables, whole grains, nuts, and fruits.

C A L C I U M : Commonly supplied in milk, cheese, leafy green vegetables, and salmon and sardines if small bones are eaten.

Although mineral loss may be significant during exercise, most authorities agree any vitamin loss, even during endurance events, is insignificant. If you eat a well-balanced diet, you will receive enough vitamins naturally for additional vitamin supplements to be unnecessary, most experts say. However, professional teams usually still give their players vitamin and mineral supplements just as added protection against any possible deficiency.

DIET NOTES

1. Because many natural vitamins and minerals are lost when food is processed or cooked in water, a good nutritional rule-of-thumb is to make sure that you eat some fresh, raw fruits and vegetables every day. Also, when possible, vegetables should be steamed or cooked quickly with as little water as possible.

2. Many athletes who seriously study nutrition

come to the conclusion that refined foods, particularly white sugar, are "dead" foods that offer almost nothing but empty calories to the body. Experts agree athletes would be far better off to avoid the likes of sugar, candy, and soda pop, and instead to get necessary calories in other foods that supply essential food elements. Reduced tooth decay is an added benefit of avoiding the sugary foods.

3. For some athletes, refined breads and cereals are in the same "dead" food category as white sugar, because a major percentage of many essential vitamins and minerals (calcium, magnesium, and potassium) is lost in the refining process and is not replaced by any "enriching" process. Recently, a South African study published in the *Journal of the American Medical Association* also suggested that overly refined foods may be largely responsible for an increase in medical ills ranging from appendicitis to heart problems and obesity. The study, which showed increases in these and other diseases as urbanized areas in Africa began consuming more refined foods instead of their traditional whole grains, said that the cereal fiber removed in refining is necessary not only for the bulk it provides "but also for its effect on the chemical and bacteriological processes that take place in the intestine."

4. Only a few top athletes in this country have been vegetarians. The most famous in recent years has been basketball's Bill Walton, and some coaches and players said that Walton seemed to be somewhat weaker and appeared to tire more quickly on the court when he took up the vegetarian diet. However, most doctors and nutritional experts agree that if he was obtaining enough protein in his diet—a major problem for vegetarians —there was probably nothing wrong with it.

Meat is the major source of protein for most American athletes, and if you cut meat from your diet, the proteins will have to be obtained elsewhere. Fish is a fine source of protein, but if fish is not acceptable to the vegetarian, other good sources include eggs, cheese and other dairy products, nuts, and soybeans.

Because protein is not an important source of energy for athletes, if a vegetarian diet includes enough carbohydrates and fats there is little likelihood that the vegetarian-athlete's endurance will suffer.

However, protein is important for muscle tissue growth and repair. Therefore, it seems likely that an athlete who is attempting to gain weight or strength through weight training, or who plays a contact sport where injuries are common, should think twice about becoming a vegetarian. Richard Wood, USC's three-time All-American linebacker, said that he felt that his strength dropped his junior year when he was following a vegetarian diet. He said he felt much stronger when he resumed his normal diet during his senior year. Randy Williams, an Olympic gold medalist in the long jump, switched to a vegetarian diet after a rash of physical ailments. However, he not only continued to train with weights but says his strength has improved with the diet. To ensure his protein intake, Williams eats eggs and fish, along with soybeans and protein supplement tablets.

5. Some athletes have such nervous stomachs that they are unable to eat the day of a game. The San Francisco 49er trainers give these players a powdered carbohydrate supplement mixed with two glasses of milk for breakfast on game days.

6. The U.S. Food and Nutrition Board recommends an average of about 2,000 calories a day for the average eighteen-to-thirty-five-year-old man. The baseball player or golfer may not require more than 2,800 daily calories, but the endurance athlete or the athlete who is training hard may consume considerably more calories than that. For example, Sherm Chavoor, whose training sessions helped produce a number of world records swim-

mers, including Mark Spitz, Mike Burton, and Debbie Meyer, gave his swimmers a diet high in fats, carbohydrates, and proteins to replace the estimated 6,000 to 7,000 calories per day some of them were burning up in the pool.

7. Highly active athletes who consume large quantities of calories during their careers often find themselves faced with weight problems after they retire from their sport because they continue to eat the same amounts while their exercise is cut back drastically. The key to weight control for any person, including old football players, is to match the food intake with energy output: if you are not very physically active, you must cut down on the amount of food you eat—it's that simple.

6. Injuries, Aches and Pains

If a man doesn't get hurt in the game, he hasn't been playing hard enough.

LARRY WILSON, *St. Louis Cardinals*

THERE IS A good chance that the athlete who is injured was playing *too* hard. At least, too hard for the shape he was in.

The athlete who is tiring and has to strain to make a play is asking for injury, regardless of whether he is playing professional football or recreational tennis.

There is a risk of injury in nearly every sport—from minor aches and pains to a potentially serious, disabling injury—but maximum, all-around (endurance, strength, flexibility) conditioning will lessen that risk, which increases with age. At the same time, the athlete who is in good shape will recover faster from any injury that does occur.

Both the fulltime and weekend athlete are likely to be concerned with preventing injuries, and also with how to recover as quickly and completely as possible. The professional athlete also has to face the prospect of playing with an injury. (Larry Wilson, the Cardinals' standout defensive safety, once played with both hands broken and in casts.) But countless athletic careers have been prematurely cut short when a player attempted to play with an injury and either made the original injury worse, or suffered another injury that might not have happened if he had been healthy.

This happens not only in professional football, where playing hurt is generally accepted as an occupational hazard, but in other sports as well, such as baseball.

Dizzy Dean was at the peak of his baseball career when he was hit in the foot by a line drive while pitching in the All-Star game. Returning to the lineup while his broken toe was still tender, Dean changed his pitching motion to avoid hurting the toe, and instead ruined his pitching arm and career.

Mickey Mantle, who hurt one knee in the 1951 World Series, said that playing when a muscle injury had not healed (and trying to keep from straining his bad knee) led to a series of problems with his other knee.

Because even a seemingly minor injury can lead to a more serious one, it makes sense that the most important injury to prevent is the *first* one.

PREVENTION

There are four basic causes of athletic injuries:

1. *Inadequate warm-up*. The player who is not *completely* loosened up before a practice or competition stands a good chance of suffering a wide range of injuries, from a sore throwing arm in baseball to strained leg muscles in virtually any fast-moving sport.

2. *Lack of flexibility*. Inadequate flexibility not only is the most common cause of muscle strains but can also lead to other injuries, including one of the most feared injuries in sports, a ruptured Achilles tendon.

3. *Poor endurance*. Most athletic injuries occur near the end of a practice or competition, when fatigue has started to set in and the athlete is straining. If an athlete lacks endurance, the time when he is vulnerable to straining already tired muscles is increased.

4. *Inadequate strength*. One effect of an injury is that surrounding muscles are weakened, thus more easily fatigued and subject to injury themselves. After a major knee injury, the leg muscles (particularly the quadriceps or upper thigh group) must be restrengthened through exercise. A lack of strength may have been a contributing factor in the original injury, but inadequate rehabilitation following an injury is almost a certain guarantee of further injury for an athlete.

Basically, the strength and flexibility exercises that have been developed to prevent the most common athletic injuries are the same exercises used in recovery from the injury after rest and treatment make rehabilitation possible.

Unfortunately, most athletes never bother with such exercises until *after* an injury. It makes better sense to do the exercises as a preventive measure against injury.

The most common athletic injuries and ailments, and the exercises designed to prevent them, include the following:

THE KNEE

The knee is the part of the body most vulnerable to serious injury in modern contact sports, simply because it was never designed to withstand the incredible strains and stresses of modern athletics, such as the impact of a fast-moving, 230-pound linebacker.

1. The single best exercise to strengthen a knee is the *leg raise,* which will develop the quadriceps muscles above the knee in the front of the thigh. The exercise can be done either with a weight machine, such as the Universal Gym, or with ankle weights (see Fig. 22). Begin with a light (two- to five-pound) weight, and do about 25 repetitions with each leg. Work up to at least 25 repetitions with from 10 to 20 percent of your body weight.

2. In the same position as the leg raise, but without weights, straighten both legs, then point your toes down and away from you as far as possible, keeping the legs stiff. Hold for about six seconds, relax, then point the toes back up and as far toward your head as possible, hold for about six seconds, relax, then press heels together, hold for about six seconds, then press big toes together, hold for about six seconds. Repeat sequence once more.

3. Both the *dead lift* and *half-squat* exercises will strengthen the quadriceps groups, and add to the support and stability of the knee.

THE ELBOW

Tennis elbow is much more common to the recreational tennis player than to the serious or fulltime tennis player because the cause is generally a poor backhand stroke, which puts a sudden, unnatural strain on the elbow. The best preventive cure for tennis elbow is simply a few hours with an instructor learning the correct stroke technique (which usually involves shifting your weight into the ball and using the racquet arm for control rather than power).

A similar elbow affliction sometimes affects baseball and football players who try to snap off a hard throw or pass, particularly without warming up. Another cause may be straining the elbow with some unfamiliar activity: Roman Gabriel blamed the sore arm that developed when he was with the Rams on a day he spent pulling crabgrass in his yard.

The chance of "thrower's elbow," as it is usually called, or tennis elbow can be greatly reduced if the muscles of the forearm are strengthened so they can better tolerate any strain or stress placed on them by a bad throw or stroke.

1. The *forearm curl* is the basic strengthening exercise for the forearm. Place your arm flat on a table so that your wrist extends over the edge. Take a dumbbell in your hand, palm up, and slowly lift your hand as high as possible without raising your forearm (it may be necessary to hold your forearm down with your other hand), then slowly lower,

The forearm curl, done both with palm up and palm down, will develop strength in the wrist as well as forearm. (PHOTOS: PONCE)

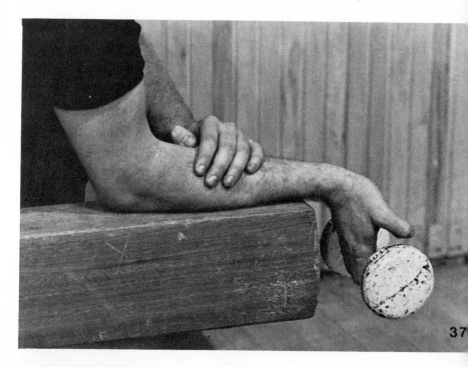

37

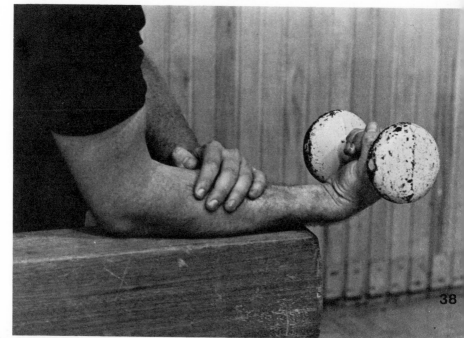

38

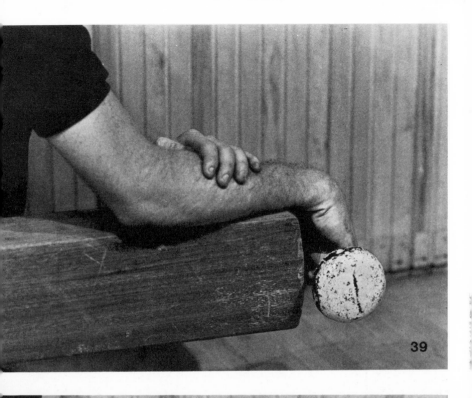

39

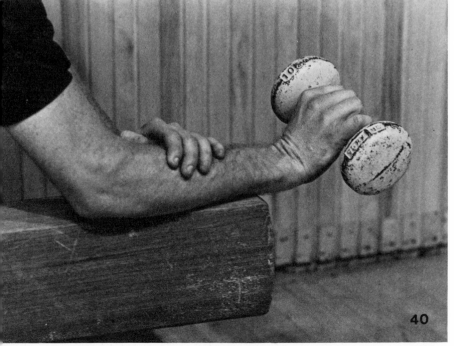

40

and repeat. After about 25 repetitions, do the same exercise again, only this time holding the dumbbell palm down, for about 25 repetitions. Begin 25 repetitions each way (palm up and palm down) with up to 10 percent of your body weight.

2. A simple but effective forearm and wrist exercise is simply squeezing a new tennis ball as hard as possible for about six seconds. Repeat 25 to 50 times. If you find a tennis ball too easy, try squeezing a rubber ball. Dodger outfielder Jimmy Wynn started squeezing a rubber ball while recovering from recent elbow surgery, and said that it made his forearm "bigger and stronger than it's ever been." This is one exercise you can do anywhere, even in your car while you are waiting for a red traffic light.

THE FOOT

The most common foot ailments affecting athletes are probably ankle sprains, Achilles tendinitis, and tennis toe.

Weak ankles cause problems not only for football players (whose ankles are usually heavily taped for support for practices as well as games) and for athletes in other sports that involve running, but also for hockey players and skiers.

1. To strengthen your ankles, do the *ankle roll*

with a barbell across your shoulders. With feet about shoulder width apart, slowly roll up onto the outer edges of your feet, then slowly roll back onto the inner edges of your feet. Repeat 10 times. You can begin this exercise with a light (25-pound) barbell. Later, if your weight program includes the military press exercise, you can use the same weight for the ankle roll.

Achilles tendinitis is an inflammation of the Achilles tendon, the cordlike tendon that attaches the calf muscles to the heel. The inflammation, which is caused by recurring strains on the tendon, if left untreated can result in a rupture or tear of the Achilles tendon.

Curiously, Achilles tendinitis, a nagging pain or tenderness at or just above the heel, often strikes distance runners who have developed strong calf muscles, as well as weekend skiers and other recreational athletes with weak calf muscles.

In the case of the runners, the reason for Achilles tendinitis usually is a lack of flexibility in the tendon, which makes it unable to handle the strains and stresses placed on it during sudden sprints, jumping, or other quick movements.

2. One exercise that will both strengthen the calf muscles and stretch the Achilles tendon is the *heel dip-and-raise*. With a light weight (25-pound)

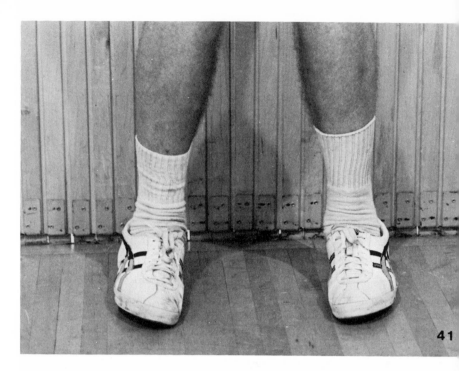

The ankle roll can be done with or without weights as an ankle strengthener.
(PHOTOS: PONCE)

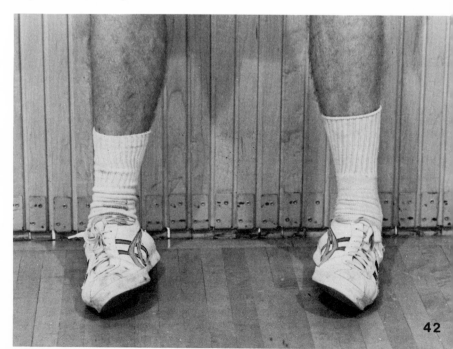

barbell on your shoulders, stand with your feet about shoulder width apart on a two-inch thick board so that your heels hang over the edge. Then slowly rise up as high as you can onto the balls of your feet, then slowly drop your heels as far as you can. Repeat about 25 times, and eventually build up to 25 repetitions with 20 to 30 percent of your body weight on the barbell.

3. Some of the flexibility exercises already described in Chapter 4, particularly the *sit reach* and others that stretch the muscles along the back of the leg, will also ease the threat of Achilles tendinitis, particularly for distance runners.

Tennis toe is a relatively new athletic injury, but it is not limited just to tennis players. In fact, Dr. Harold Roth, who presented the first medical paper on the problem, first guessed at the cause of the ailment while watching a Los Angeles Laker basketball game. He noticed that the newer European-designed tennis shoes the players were wearing had tremendous gripping power in the sole tread. The increased traction combined with the narrower toe sections of the new sneakers to jam the athlete's large toes against the front of the shoes. The result is sometimes a painful swelling and bleeding under the toenail. The cure, however, is simplicity itself: If you play a sport that de-

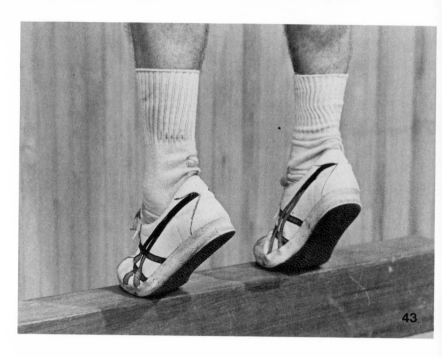

43

The heel dip-and-raise is another exercise that can be done without weights to increase flexibility in the Achilles tendon (during the dip). With weights, the exercise will develop strength in the calf muscles in the lower leg. (PHOTOS: PONCE)

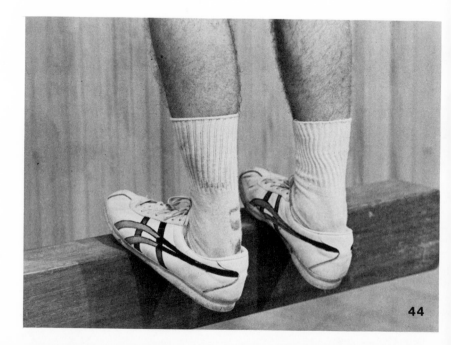

44

mands quick stops, such as tennis and basketball, wear a tennis shoe that offers plenty of room in the toe area.

THE SHOULDER

Most shoulder ailments, including bursitis and tendinitis, like most elbow ailments, are caused by poor athletic form during a movement involving the shoulder, such as throwing a javelin or baseball, or spiking a volleyball. Again, as with the elbow, a gradual warming up before play is essential.

Some of the basic weight-training exercises presented in Chapter 3, including the *bench press* and the *military press* will help strengthen the shoulder.

1. Another basic shoulder exercise is the *arm raise*. With a dumbbell in each hand, slowly raise your arms—keeping them stiff—out from each side of your body, hold for about five seconds, and then slowly lower to your sides again. Repeat 25 times. Then repeat the exercise, only this time lift your arms directly in front of you, hold for five seconds, and then lower. Do 25 repetitions. This is one exercise that generally requires a very light (two to five pound) weight in the beginning. If you have adjustable dumbbells, start by using just the bar alone, or hold one of the lighter weight plates in each hand.

2. A good preactivity stretching exercise for the shoulders is the *finger grip*. If you are unable to grip your fingers, try to reach as far as possible each day until you can, but only to the point of pain. When you are able to touch or grip your fingers, slowly pull back both shoulders at the same time, again only to the point of pain.

THE BACK

Most back pains and muscle strains in the back can be relieved through a combination of flexibility and strength exercises.

Weak abdominal ("gut") muscles are the major cause for most common back pains. Abdominal muscles are one of the major muscle groups supporting the spine, and if the abdominals are weak, the other muscle groups tend to "overcompensate" or "oversupport" the spine, causing improper spine alignment and pain.

The best conditioner for abdominals is the *bent leg sit-up*. UCLA's Jim Bush says he does about 10 bent leg sit-ups any time he feels his back starting to hurt.

Straight leg sit-ups involve the use of the hip flexor muscles, while the bent leg sit-ups concentrate the exercise on the abdominals, particularly when the feet are not held down.

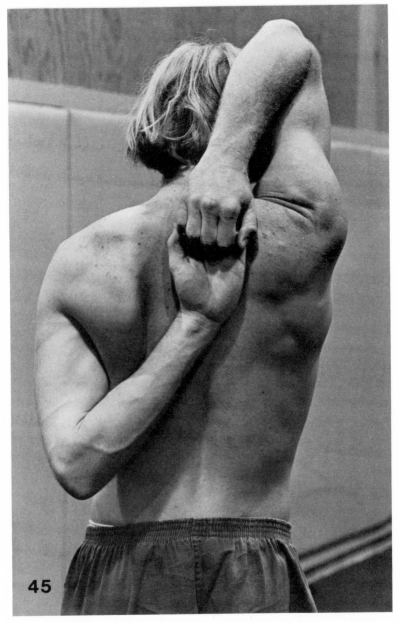

45

The finger grip is a good exercise for increasing shoulder flexibility. Try to grip fingers (many athletes are unable even to touch their fingers when first beginning this exercise) and then push shoulders backward; hold for five seconds, then push forward and hold again.

Always try to do sit-ups on a soft or padded surface, and avoid jerking up that might cause a muscle strain in the back or abdominals. Instead roll up from the floor into the sit-up.

TREATMENT AND RECOVERY

Always remember that pain is a warning signal from the body.

If the pain from an injury or ailment is severe, or if a minor pain persists, consult a physician. Playing with pain may be required of some professional athletes, but it is the surest way of making a minor injury worse.

The professional athlete who suffers a knee injury is almost certain to be examined by trainers and physicians immediately. If required, surgery is likely to be completed in the next day or two, because prompt surgery (in the case of ligament damage) is generally more successful than that done later.

However, the weekend athlete who feels a "pop" in his knee during a tennis match or a pick-up basketball game often does not see a doctor at all. Later, if the pain subsides, he will probably convince himself he wasn't hurt that badly in the first place and, with weakened muscles as a result of the injury, go back to his athletic activity with a much greater risk of further injury.

What should you do after you are hurt until you are able to contact a doctor? Most coaches have traditionally felt the basic treatment for almost any injury is *rest,* in the belief that minor injuries will heal themselves and more serious injuries won't be made worse.

However, the Rams under Gary Tuthill have found more success with letting an injured player exercise gradually and carefully as soon as he can. A player with a muscle pull, for example, may be encouraged to jog a little the day after an injury. Tuthill says it is important not to push the player beyond what he is capable of for fear of making the injury worse. But at the same time, too much inactivity after an injury can lead to atrophied muscles and a longer recovery time, he says.

There is almost unanimous agreement among most professional trainers that the first treatment for nearly every athletic injury should be applications of ice.

Chuck Krpata, head trainer of the San Francisco 49ers and holder of a master's degree in physical therapy, points out that there are eight times as many "cold receptors" as "heat receptors" in the body. Not only is treatment with ice the best way to prevent swelling and hemorrhaging, but the ice treatment also has a more lasting effect than heat treatments.

Sandy Koufax, who was one of the first pitchers to begin the practice of soaking his throwing arm in ice after every game, and Bill Walton, who puts ice on his knees right after he leaves the basketball court, are just two of the better known athletes who have relied on ice treatments.

After the initial ice treatments, many trainers alternate heat and ice treatments during the next several days.

A guide to exercising while recovering from an injury, Tuthill says, is "do what you can only to the point of pain."

If you have a leg injury, swimming or bicycling may help you maintain your endurance conditioning if you are unable to run.

But with any serious injury, advice on what type of exercise you can do during recovery should come from a doctor.

7. The Weekend Athlete

I F   Y O U   are not presently getting vigorous exercise (at least 30 minutes to one hour) three to four days a week, you are shortchanging your basic health needs—to say nothing of falling short of the conditioning necessary for athletic activity.

But the typical "weekend athlete" often sits around his office and home all week long, and then on Saturday grabs his tennis racquet and goes out and plays some fast singles until he is ready to drop, with the belief that pushing himself to exhaustion was good evidence that he got enough "exercise" for the week.

That kind of infrequent but intense exercise does far more harm than good.

The jogger who collapses after a run and the

tennis player who suffers a heart attack during a weekend tournament are usually victims of too little—and too much—exercise.

Too much exercise can be dangerous, even fatal, if you have not been exercising enough to allow your body to adapt gradually to the increased exertion.

Furthermore, it is the regular, steady diet of exercise, not just occasional, strenuous exercise, that increases fitness by improving the efficiency of the respiratory and cardiovascular systems.

So if you exercise only one or two days a week (whether those days happen to be Saturday, Sunday, or Tuesday), you should exercise lightly, or even not exercise at all, rather than exercise strenuously and exhaust yourself on a haphazard, occasional basis.

But because regular exercise is so beneficial to all-around health, you would be much wiser to build a regular exercise or conditioning program around your sport activities.

That doesn't mean you have to run or do 15 minutes of boring calisthenics each day.

If you enjoy running, then run. For the amount of time spent, it is the handiest, most efficient method to get the basic conditioning you need for good health. If you run—not jog (see Chapter 2)

—for 20 to 30 minutes a day, three days a week; or 12 to 15 minutes a day, five times a week, most authorities agree you are getting enough exercise to meet general health needs and to maintain a basic level of conditioning fitness.

But if you don't like to run, chances are even if you start a running program, you probably will quit it fairly soon.

The key to conditioning is to find activities and exercises you enjoy so that you will stay with them on a regular basis.

If you like, or think you might like, playing tennis, give it a try. Depending on how you play the game, tennis can be a good conditioning exercise. (If you play doubles, or if you just stand in one spot and make an effort to hit only the balls that come right to you, you won't benefit much in the way of conditioning exercise.)

If you play an hour or more of fast-moving singles five days a week, you should be getting enough conditioning exercise from tennis alone. Now, you may not have time for tennis five days a week. However, if you play tennis twice a week and also get some other exercise (running, swimming, bicycling, skipping rope, or some other sport) at other times during the week, you are likely to be meeting your endurance or conditioning needs.

You should also be able to meet those needs with the following:

Swimming (nonstop): 30 minutes, three times a week; or 15 to 20 minutes, five times a week.

Rope skipping: 15 minutes, five times a week.

Nordic (*cross-country*) *skiing:* 30 to 40 minutes, three times a week; or 20 to 25 minutes, five times a week.

Basketball, football, handball, hockey, alpine (*downhill*) *skiing, soccer, surfing, volleyball* (*two-man*): 60 minutes, four times a week; or 45 minutes, five times a week.

Tennis (*singles*), *volleyball* (*six-man*): 60 minutes, five times a week.

Golf (*18 holes*), *walking* (*three miles in 45 minutes*): six times a week.

If you haven't been exercising regularly, you should begin slowly, at an easy, comfortable pace, no matter what sport or activity you are pursuing. For example, if necessary begin the running program with about 10 minutes of jogging-walking.

The most comprehensive approach yet developed for meeting basic endurance levels is the "aerobics" exercise programs devised by Dr. Kenneth Cooper. The programs are age-adjusted and offer a week-by-week guide to building endurance gradually through a variety of physical activities, including walking, running, swimming, and bicycling.

However, endurance is not the only area of physical fitness that is important to the weekend or occasional athlete.

Weight training and other strength exercises are largely unnecessary for the weekend athlete. Two exercises that are a good idea for any active person, however, are sit-ups and push-ups.

Bent leg sit-ups, done without anyone holding your feet down, are the best guarantee against low back pains that are the result of weak abdominal muscles, while push-ups are a quick, easy way to maintain basic upper body muscle tone. Doing just 20 of each exercise every day takes less than two minutes, and is well worth the time.

Flexibility exercises are also worthwhile for the weekend athlete—particularly for those who play more physical or active sports.

The businessman who plays basketball at noon each day suffers just as much pain from an injury as the professional athlete. And, depending on his line of work, being disabled can be almost as costly.

Some injuries are unavoidable. But many, including most muscle strains and pulls, can be prevented with regular stretching exercises, which also help to ease the stiffness that follows the Sunday touch football game or the annual weekend tennis tournament.

8. The Female Athlete

THE EXPANSION of programs for women athletes at both the collegiate and high school level is just one indication of the remarkable growth women's athletics have undergone in the past few years. And with the greater acceptance of women as athletes, more and more female athletes are turning to conditioning to find a competitive edge.

While the physiology of women is, of course, different from the physiology of men, the basic training methods are the same for both female and male athletes. The basic difference between the conditioning programs of men and women is that male athletes have been training at much more intense levels than female athletes.

When a female athlete begins to equal the training intensity of male athletes, she is usually a world-class competitor. A case in point is Francie Larrieu, the United States' premier female distance runner, who runs about 70 to 80 miles a week and works out with male runners during daily training sessions at the UCLA track. Still, Larrieu concedes that "even on my best days" she couldn't beat the male runners she trains with.

Part of the reason may be simply because women have a higher percentage of fat than men; a study of college-age athletes by Dr. Jack Wilmore of UC Davis showed the body weight of the female athletes was 25 percent fat, compared with only 15 percent for the male athletes.

Dr. Joan Ullyot of the Pacific Medical Center said a recent study showed women's higher fat content can be an advantage in long distance running. Noting that only enough glycogen can be stored in muscle tissue to last about two hours, or about 20 miles of running, Dr. Ullyot said that after the 20-mile mark, when muscles have to rely on energy stored in fat, women often start running more efficiently than men. A runner herself, Dr. Ullyot was among the top finishers in the 26-mile International Women's Marathon in Germany in 1974. (It should also be noted that most top male distance runners have trained to where their fat content is less than 10 percent.)

But for most athletic efforts, body fat is a disadvantage, and by comparison with male athletes, the female athlete suffers for her higher fat content.

Although the endurance of the woman athlete can begin to approach the endurance levels of men (Larrieu's times for the mile, for example, are better than the vast majority of male high school runners, and approach those of most college milers), the difference in strength is the most striking difference between men and women athletes. A basic reason, researchers say, is that testosterone, a male hormone, gives men a greater potential for muscle mass than women.

To overcome this strength disadvantage, an increasing number of female athletes are taking up weight training.

Several studies by Wilmore and Dr. C. Harmon Brown, California State University at Hayward, of women (ranging from teen-age national track champions to untrained college-age females) showed weight training led to average strength gains of from about 20 to 40 percent.

Wilmore noted that the greatest strength improvement among women was evident in the upper body, suggesting that even a nonathletic woman exercises her legs in her daily routines, such as walking.

Despite the significant strength gains, the women in the studies showed little increase in muscle bulk—which Dr. Brown attributed to lack of testosterone. Wilmore suggests that, for this reason, women can use weight training to develop strength without worrying about developing a heavily muscled body.

Another Wilmore study found that in a 10-week, three-workouts-per-week test, the women involved showed strength gains of from 20 to 50 percent, while at the same time slimming the waist, hips, and buttocks, and without experiencing any weight gain.

Weight training has become common practice among many female track and field athletes, particularly those involved in the strength events, such as the discus and shotput.

A woman athlete who wants increased strength but is worried about adding too much muscle bulk can work to increase the speed of her weight training workouts rather than to increase the weight overload. For example, after 8 to 12 weeks of weight training, she should stop increasing the weight in the different exercises, and instead try to work at completing her normal (say 30-minute) routine in 25 minutes, and then 20 minutes. If she maintains the same weight for the exercises and continues with the same workout routine (number of sets and repetitions), she'll keep her muscle tone without any increase in muscle size, according to Frank Egenhoff, weight training coach for the San Francisco 49ers.

Flexibility, the other main component of athletic fitness, is just as important for women as men. But possibly because of their general lack of intensive training, most women seem to be somewhat more flexible than men. Therefore, flexibility is the one area of athletic conditioning in which women do not have to start at a disadvantage to men.

9. Some Final Notes

A T   W H A T   A G E   should   an   athlete   stop training?

Most athletes, including the large majority of football, baseball, and basketball players, give up their favorite sports at a relatively early age. However, for general health reasons an athlete, or any other individual, should find some other ways (a new sport, bicycling or running) of staying in shape.

An example of what the "elderly" athlete is capable of was Jack LaLanne's two-mile swim from Alcatraz Island to San Francisco's Fishermen's Wharf on his sixtieth birthday. With the ocean water temperature in the 50s, LaLanne made the swim towing a 1,000-pound boat, with his *hands and feet bound*. To prepare himself for the ordeal, LaLanne spent 90 minutes a day weight lifting, 30 minutes a day swimming, and 30 minutes a day running. He also spent up to an hour a day just sitting in an ice-filled bathtub in an effort to get used to the cold water.

Another example is Monty Montgomery, who last year at sixty-eight ran a 26-mile Santa Barbara marathon in 2 hours, 56 minutes—almost a half hour better than any other man his age has ever done. And Montgomery, who has been active all his life, didn't begin running competitively until he was sixty-three.

In that same marathon race, finishing in 3 hours, 59 minutes, was sixty-two-year-old Bud Robinson. What was remarkable about Robinson's performance was that only eight months before he had undergone open heart surgery to have a coronary artery bypass operation. Robinson's doctors believe that if he hadn't been physically active (he started running when he was fifty-nine), his heart wouldn't have been strong enough to survive the attack that prompted the operation.

However, at the same time, it is probably safe to say that no two athletes, coaches, or trainers have ever agreed on exactly what is the best training for athletic fitness. A case in point is the "Six

Rules for a Happy Life" suggested by Satchel Paige:

1. Avoid fried meats, which angry up the blood.
2. If your stomach disputes you, lie down and pacify it with cool thoughts.
3. Keep the juices flowing by jangling around gently as you move.
4. Go lightly on the vices, such as carrying on in society. The social ramble ain't restful.
5. Avoid running at all times.
6. Don't look back, something may be gaining on you.

Paige, with his incredible pitching talents, may have been able to follow his Rule No. 5 and still be successful. It is the opinion of leading coaches and trainers that most career athletes today can't afford that luxury, at least not without worrying about his Rule No. 6.

Dewey Schurman

Dewey Schurman, a graduate of the University of California, Santa Barbara, is a staff writer for the Santa Barbara *News-Press*. He lives in Montecito, California, with his wife and two children. He is the author of a book on volleyball skills.